PRAISE FOR KEEP

"Heart-tugging stories, sage ███████████████████ make this a must-have book for ████████████ rom PTSD or any other trauma. With masterful writing, the authors help the reader let go of the past, live in the present and, perhaps most important of all, look forward to the future."

—Allen Klein, bestselling author of *The Healing Power of Humor* and *You Can't Ruin My Day*

"This book offers real stories and a path to authentic emotional healing for people recovering from past hurts and traumatic events. Writing with hope and compassion, the authors guide the reader through an actionable stepwise process of gaining their life back after traumatic experiences and keeping the emotional pain in the past—for good!"

—Helen Odessky, PsyD, author of *Stop Anxiety from Stopping You*

"Millions of people suffer from PTSD which can dramatically impact their lives. The self-healing process mapped out in *Keep Pain in the Past* is based on decades of successful treatment of patients and offers help and hope to those who need it. With this remarkable remedy, readers can go from surviving to thriving."

—Dr. John Duffy, author of *The Available Parent*; also podcasts on WGN Radio's "BETTER" show

"*Keep Pain in the Past* is a well-thought-out tome of helpful, step-by-step tools for healing from physical and emotional trauma. Authors Cortman and Walden present questions for the reader to ask himself or herself at the end of each chapter and provide suggestions that are sensible and real for one to step out of PTSD and to step up to his or her brighter future."

—KJ Landis, author of *Happy Healthy You*

"Individuals suffering from drug and alcohol or other addictions, or from anxiety, depression, resentment, and compulsive behavior, as well as those having difficulty moving on from bad experiences, can greatly benefit from the knowledge and practical exercises in this book."

—Calvina Fay, executive director, Drug Free America Foundation, Inc.

"Time may not heal all wounds, but a powerful process can. I'm so grateful to the authors of *Keep Pain in the Past* for restoring hope that trauma can be healed without years of psychotherapy. Each wounded heart is longing to be whole again. This book is the perfect companion for that journey."

—MK Mueller, author of *8 to Great*

"The work Dr. Chris Cortman is doing in the field of trauma recovery is some of the most important work being done today. In *Keep Pain in the Past*, he shares the compelling stories of people he has helped using a simple (though not easy) five-step framework. Through these stories, helpful writing prompts, and other detailed tools and resources, readers see what is actually possible in regards to recovering from trauma (whether with a capital T or a small t), and can begin to attend to their own recovery. I am looking forward to employing 'The Fritz' in my own ongoing personal work!"

—Karen C.L. Anderson, author of *Difficult Mothers, Adult Daughters: A Guide for Separation, Liberation & Inspiration*

KEEP
PAIN IN
THE PAST

For permission requests, please contact the publisher at:

Mango Publishing Group
2850 Douglas Road, 3rd Floor
Coral Gables, FL 33134 U.S.A.
info@mango.bz

For special orders, quantity sales, course adoptions and corporate sales, please email the publisher at sales@mango.bz. For trade and wholesale sales, please contact Ingram Publisher Services at:
customer.service@ingramcontent.com or +1.800.509.4887.

Keep Pain in the Past: Getting Over Trauma, Grief and the Worst That's Ever Happened to You

Library of Congress Cataloging
ISBN: (p) 978-1-63353-810-8, (e) 978-1-63353-811-5
Library of Congress Control Number: 2018952275
BISAC—PSY022040—PSYCHOLOGY / Psychopathology / Post-Traumatic Stress Disorder (PTSD)

Printed in the United States of America.

KEEP PAIN IN THE PAST

GETTING OVER TRAUMA, GRIEF AND THE WORST THAT'S EVER HAPPENED TO YOU

DR. CHRIS CORTMAN & DR. JOSEPH WALDEN

Mango Publishing

CORAL GABLES, FL

 mango

This book is dedicated to everyone who's been told, "Time heals all wounds," but it didn't. It's also dedicated to people who were told, "It's called PTSD, and there is no cure, so you just have to live with it." Let me not forget those who were told that, "There is no such thing as multiple personality, you're making that up for attention." And, of course, it's for people who were sexually assaulted, molested, raped, sold, abused, and then when you bravely told someone, you weren't believed.

This book is for all of you who have been abandoned, betrayed, neglected, threatened, beaten, terrorized, bullied, cheated on, swindled, scammed, conned, rejected, or never picked for the basketball team. It's for you who have come forth and told your story, and especially for you who as yet have not. This book is for anyone willing to hope and believe one more time. This book is for you.

CONTENTS

Chapter One

Treating Trauma; What If We Already Have the Answers We Need to Heal?

"Time passages. There's something back here that you left behind. Oh, time passages. Buy me a ticket on the last train home tonight."

—Al Stewart

Is Anyone Living in the Now?

"Are you at peace with everything that has ever happened to you?" I asked my waitress, wanting to satisfy my curiosity about how someone outside a clinical setting might respond. "Are you living completely in the present, looking forward?"

"Wow, I thought when you said you had a couple of questions, you were going to ask if you could replace the fries with soup without paying extra," said the server. "But to answer your questions, no, I'm not over my past, is anyone? And for what it's worth, it's an extra dollar to replace the fries with today's soup of the day, chicken noodle."

Now ask yourself the same question (about your life, not the soup). Have you put the painful events and traumas of your life into a healthy place? Are you free of regret, resentment, and painful, intrusive memories? If you answered yes, you can stop reading right now. You don't need this book, since you're living a fully realized, highly successful life in the here and now.

Most people, though, aren't in this enviable position. Your life is compromised in some way by a trauma from your past. You may not be conscious of it, but that trauma weighs on your like an anchor, dragging down your career, your relationships, and your life. That's the bad news. The good news is that regardless of what you have experienced, you can take your pain in the past, process and digest it, find meaning in your suffering, and champion the trauma, once and for all.

A case in point is Jim, one of my clients. Jim is an extreme case—I hope that whatever bad things have happened in your life are nowhere near as bad as what happened to Jim. He was suffering from severe post-traumatic stress disorder (PTSD), and I must warn you that his story is disturbing.

Your particular pain in the past may not be as extreme, but all emotional trauma has similar symptoms. Using Jim's story, I will highlight the common trauma symptoms and how they can ravage a life if not treated properly. Also, I aim to provide you with hope: if Jim can be treated effectively, anyone can be.

After telling Jim's story, I'll provide some questions that will help you think about your own therapeutic experiences related to what Jim experienced. Then, I'll examine six different perspectives (five scientific and one religious) that have contributed to my understanding of how to treat trauma successfully. Finally, I'll compare what I believe to be unhelpful treatments with my approach.

An Evolving Tragedy

One day, just before Christmas some forty five years ago, Jim was enjoying a brisk Connecticut afternoon on the river near his house with his two sons, eight-year-old Jim Jr. and five-year-old Kevin. The boys were elated to pile out of Jim's old Country Squire and eager to go skating.

The river was solid, and the new skates—Christmas presents opened early, without mom's knowledge—fit perfectly. Kevin told his dad and his brother that this was bound to be the "best day ever!"

And so, it was, until his boys reached the midway point of the river. Jim heard the cracking of the ice while he was setting up a hockey net on the near side. Before he could react, he saw the terror on their faces just before they were swallowed up by the icy waters. Jim speed skated to the opening and dove head first into the hole into which his children had plummeted. He couldn't find them because the currents had taken the children hundreds of yards downstream. Ultimately, no one found them until three days later.

As you can imagine, Jim and his wife, Ruth, were devastated but committed to surviving their horror. Though Jim felt horrible—he had committed the unforgivable sin of allowing his children to perish—he knew that for Ruth's sake, he had to try to get past this tragedy. They went to Hawaii in an attempt to "escape" what had happened.

That was a well-intentioned mistake. Tragedies are not confined to the zip code in which they occur. Images of the drowned children haunted them, even in the paradise of Hawaii. It was the last time Jim and Ruth attempted a vacation. They needed to devise a better, more realistic solution to their grief. They decided to have another child. Michael was sweet, intelligent, and extremely affectionate, but he couldn't fulfill the expectations imposed upon his tiny shoulders. He was unable to eliminate the memory of his brothers.

Michael's birth made Jim even more conscious of his dead sons. He adored Michael but couldn't bear to let him get close emotionally. "Christ, what if God took him, too?" was his thought. So he distanced himself from his baby boy by preoccupying himself with work. Ironically, this made Jim feel more disgusted with himself and reinforced his "worst father" internal image. Ruth observed this silently. She knew Jim was sinking but didn't know how to help him.

At Ruth's insistence, Jim sought psychiatric help, but the antidepressants did little to make Jim care about life again. Soon, he stopped taking them. He didn't blame Dr. Evans; how could a pill make his life any better? Did they have a pill that could bring his boys back? He did blame God, however: "You sacrificed your son, but took two of mine." At times, he thought his silent rage and blasphemous thoughts would assure him a spot in Hell, but then again, how could Hell be any worse than this? Besides, if anyone deserved to be in Hell, it was the negligent father who'd allowed his kids to drown.

Jim did find respite, or more accurately, distraction, on the job. He worked tirelessly as an auto mechanic. He loved cars almost as much as he loved motorcycles, and he put in twelve-hour days routinely. He knew he was shortchanging Michael, but he rationalized his long work days.

He found other distractions, namely motorcycle riding and drinking binges. When Jim resided in the darkest of places, he combined the two. Something about riding at 110 miles per hour (with Johnny Walker Red as copilot) could make Jim Jr. and Kevin all but fade away. He also recognized how dangerous this behavior was and how he was half hoping that a fatal accident might obliterate his emotional pain.

Jim settled on alcohol as the best alternative to suicide—that and a compulsive work ethic. He did as well as he could with Michael, participated in Boy

Scouts, and even co-managed his little league team one year. But there was no ice skating, ever.

I began working with Jim forty-five years after the tragedy. He was suffering from chronic depression, with symptoms like "anhedonia" (deriving little joy from activities that once provided happiness and contentment) and dysphoria (low mood). He also was afflicted with insomnia—four uninterrupted hours was a good night's sleep—and he was tortured by nihilistic or "what's the point in life?" type thinking and horrible self-contempt ("They died on my watch!"). There was also a generalized anxiety—Jim called it his racing motor—and chronic fatigue. With more than just symptoms of depression and anxiety, Jim met the criteria for a common psychiatric diagnosis known as Post-Traumatic Stress Disorder (PTSD).

Despite his best efforts to run away from the past, Jim was haunted by intrusive recollections of the traumatic event, "Just how many times do I have to see that helpless look on Kevin's face before he plunges into the water?" There were also flashbacks of the headfirst dive, the frantic calls for help, and the sleepless nights before the bodies were found.

Like almost all PTSD sufferers, Jim avoided any reminders of the tragedy; no New York Rangers season tickets, no desire to be around families (since his was irretrievably broken), no anniversary of the death, no birthdays, no mention of the boys, and for God's sake, no talking about the event! Holidays were intolerable, and family members or friends who were likely to offer consolation or "lame advice" were to be avoided at all costs. "Ruth could see 'em if she wanted to, but I wasn't going." Avoidance also meant moving to another town, away from the neighbors who knew him and knew what had happened, away from his church, and away from that godforsaken river. And avoidance was the reason Jim drank himself to oblivion. Before the accident, he had been a social drinker; afterwards, he employed the hard stuff to "transport myself to another reality."

He also convinced Ruth to move to Florida, in large part because of the fiercely negative connotations ice and cold had for him. Perhaps the most serious repercussion of Jim's emotional trauma, however, was that it made him hypervigilant, especially with Michael. Only when Ruth protested that Jim was overly controlling did he finally back off. But that meant distancing himself from Michael, not learning to give him appropriate space to grow up. As a result, it was sometimes hard, Jim admits, to decide which version of himself was worse: overprotective, controlling Jim, or the distant, uncaring man who spent nights on the recliner with Johnny Walker Red.

Before Jim arrived in my Florida office, he had been to four mental health professionals over the years, but never went to more than three or four sessions with any of them. He was not about to try antidepressants again; "When I explained that to these shrinks, it looked like they were lost in the fear of 'what do we do now?'"

Jim was pleased that I didn't care if he took antidepressants. "They aren't the answer to helping you heal from your losses."

"You mean there's a way to heal from this?"

"Actually, yes. I'd like to help you to get a place of peace, if you are willing to follow a plan with me. Healing requires action—there are things we need to do in order for you to recover from your losses."

I explained PTSD to him using the following analogy: In some ways, your mind is kind of like the stomach. Whatever has not been digested may come back up on you. Of course, while the stomach can only keep food undigested for eight to ten hours, the mind can hold undigested material for decades without ever eliminating it. Healing requires the ability to release the painful material to regain any semblance of peace. I told him I wanted to help him release his trauma once and for all.

∞

Let's leave Jim's treatment for the time being. (I promise we will return to it later in the book.) But for now, let's explore his many years of (unnecessary) suffering. Why was it that the mental health professionals he saw never helped him?

Societal bias has favored a medical model of treatment for most everything that ails us, including symptoms of PTSD and other forms of emotional trauma. Doctors have prescribed antidepressants for symptoms of depression and anxiety, tranquilizers and sedatives for insomnia, and mood stabilizers to address emotionally instability. If all else fails, antipsychotic medication has been prescribed as "a glue to keep it together." Unfortunately, an abundance of research demonstrates that medications at best mask symptoms of PTSD and at worst create numerous and often debilitating side effects. The U.S. Department of Veterans Affairs[2] states that "Trauma-focused psychotherapies are more efficacious than pharmacotherapy and are strongly recommended treatments for PTSD." (Jeffreys, M. 2017) A booklet provided by the National Center for PTSD[3] for veterans seeking treatment says, "Medications can treat PTSD symptoms alone or with therapy—but only therapy treats the underlying cause of your symptoms. If you treat your PTSD symptoms only with medication, you'll need to keep taking it for it to keep working." (National Center for PTSD, 2018,) The VA, which is the biggest provider of trauma treatment, and National Center for PTSD, which is the biggest researcher of PTSD, both agree that medication never helps the underlying cause of the symptoms—the unresolved trauma. In fact, by successfully masking symptoms, medications may actually interfere with effective treatment, as clients may settle for a treatment that distances them from their emotional pain. Antidepressants and tranquilizers are notorious for masking emotional pain (emotional anesthesia), although they can prevent people from disintegrating into a puddle of tears. Most people enjoy that feature of antidepressants, and they often conclude that masking the pain is as good as it's going to get.

Ironically, one of the prominent symptoms of PTSD is avoidance, as noted above in Jim's story. Consequently, let me state this as boldly as possible (I'll even use bold print): **Prescribing only psychotropic medication without healing psychotherapy may contribute to the client avoiding the problem, rather than addressing and healing it! In fact, while I'm out of a controversial limb, "medication only" treatment for unresolved emotional trauma can be tantamount to enabling the client to remain stuck in the symptoms of PTSD.**

Medicating clients' suffering without addressing the place where they are stuck in the pain of the past supports them in remaining mired there without having to address and resolve the underlying issue(s). Moreover, if clients are numb enough to function (albeit unhappily), they can avoid facing their pain head-on, which is a requirement of effective psychological treatment. After all, people don't tend to present for psychological treatment unless they are in crisis mode—in layman's terms, not unless they're coming apart at the seams. Alas, as the great Dr. James Framo[4], a former professor of mine, used to say, "People don't change unless it's too painful not to."

If medication separates people from their pain, they are less likely to address their underlying issues. Allow me a crude but hopefully accurate analogy: If a client has a large, unpassable kidney stone trapped in the ureter, the pain motivates the client to find a doctor who can remove it. But if allowed generous amounts of opioids, that same client may postpone (i.e., avoid) the surgery indefinitely, as long as the pain is manageable. If the stone isn't removed from the ureter, though, it will do long-term damage.

I'm not opposed to medication; I'm only opposed to medication that prevents the root cause of emotional trauma from being addressed. The psychological community appears to be equally culpable in Jim's forty-five years of misery. Let me illustrate: At a recent professional psychology conference, I listened to a capable presenter discuss the two "leading treatments for PTSD." She shared that Eye Movement Desensitization and Reprocessing (EMDR) and Prolonged Exposure (PE) were the best treatments we had at this time.

I sat there stewing, knowing she was wrong. But how could she have been so unaware of the much more effective alternatives to treating emotional trauma? Here's how. Various psychological schools and practitioners, past and present, offer an abundance of training, research, and theories on everything from psychological development to personality theory to effective treatments for psychological disorders. There is no one paradigm or model from which to draw. Psychologists emerge from their training with the theories and styles that best fit each practitioner. That only makes sense, but it also guarantees that if you enter six psychologists' offices, you are likely to receive six different (albeit potentially similar) therapeutic styles and treatment plans to address the very same presenting issues.

One therapist, for instance, may operate from the belief that you the client have suffered enough trauma already, so the last thing you need to do is revisit the scene of the crime. What the client needs instead are coping tools. This well-intentioned approach, though, may help you cope but not thrive. You may be able to maintain a relationship and a job but probably never be able to enjoy either. Until you make peace with the pain in your past, you will never do much more than cope.

Other therapists try to help you to rethink the traumatic event. These therapists might have tried to convince Jim that he'd had about three minutes to locate his two sons, rescue them from the icy water, and revive them, and that given the impossibility of doing so within this time frame, he should free himself from his guilt. They would provide him with other types of useful and realistic information to alter his beliefs about the trauma. This might help Jim to some extent, but it wouldn't allow him to release the intrusive attacks of the undigested trauma.

Some psychologists believe in using highly specialized approaches, such as eye movement desensitization and reprocessing techniques (EMDR), which requires clients to visualize the trauma while watching an object such as a pencil move back and forth. While the visualization of the trauma is necessary for healing to occur, the eye movement is extraneous and completely unnecessary. What is paramount, however, is the need to release the traumatic event permanently, which in my opinion, EMDR does not accomplish effectively.

And there are therapists who base their treatment on a behavioral principle called "flooding", which employs a technique called prolonged exposure (PE) where clients are asked to revisualize and re-experience the trauma continuously until they are habituated (i.e., stop responding emotionally) to it. While remembering the traumatic event fully is important (as you will see, it's step one of the Fritz), simply remembering it over and over again is unnecessarily torturous, forcing people to relive the biggest horror of their lives repeatedly. This is cruel and unusual punishment, especially given that a single return to the trauma is all that is required to find peace with the intrusive recollections and stop the nightmares.

ASSESS YOUR OWN TREATMENT

As you read about these various treatment types, at least one of them may have struck a chord with you because of your own journey. It's worth assessing that particular form of therapy (or those therapies) and what went wrong; or what failed to go sufficiently right so that you could now be living a life free of the effects of your trauma.

Take a look at the following questions and think about your answers:

- What type of therapy did you use? What method did your therapist employ (assuming he or she disclosed this method), or from what therapeutic school of thought did your therapist develop his or her method?

- How long were you in therapy? Did you stop for a particular reason?

- Are you a serial therapy-seeker? How many different therapists or types of therapy have you had?

- Have you been prescribed any medications to help you deal with the problems stemming from your trauma? What are the medications, and how effective have they been, both in addressing the short-term symptoms as well as in helping you heal and lead a fulfilling, successful life?

- How much work on your issues have you done on your own? Did your therapist suggest you should be working on healing outside of his/her office? Did your therapist give you any tools or techniques to use on your own?

- How has the emotional trauma you suffered affected your life negatively? Has it negatively affected you in terms of your careers, relationships, moods, or ability to enjoy life? Has therapy helped you deal successfully with any of these problems, especially in the long term?

ANALYSIS: PUTTING YOUR THERAPY ON THE COUCH

- *What type of therapy did you use? What method did your therapist employ (assuming he or she disclosed this method), or from what "school" of therapy did your therapist develop his or her method?*

If you don't know what type of therapy or school of thought your therapist uses, you're not alone. Your therapist may not have divulged this information to you for a variety of reasons—he or she may not have found it therapeutically beneficial, for instance. It's also possible that your therapist does not endorse a particular approach or theoretical construct to treat trauma. In either case, as a client, you're in the dark, and you shouldn't be.

- *How long were you in therapy? Did you stop for a particular reason?*

You may have been in therapy for many years and continued to wait for it to work. You may have also tried therapy for a short period of time and quit because you weren't seeing any results. In either case, the lesson learned is that time is not a predictor of effectiveness. Every client is different, and it takes longer to heal some emotional traumas than others. That said, the right therapy should work relatively quickly.

- *Are you a serial therapy-seeker? How many different therapists or types of therapy have you had?*

Bouncing around from one therapist to another is incredibly frustrating, and if this has been your experience, I apologize on behalf of our profession. The odds are that if you've seen multiple therapists without much success, then you probably didn't feel safe or heard when you were in therapy. With Jim, I assured him that effective trauma treatment existed for his particular issues and that healing was possible, and I did this in our very first session. Without believing a therapist "gets" what you've been through and that (s) he can help you, you won't feel safe or heard and will leave, usually sooner rather than later. Maybe therapies you've experienced have been focused on coping instead of healing. Remember, many therapists focus on coping rather than healing, as such therapists don't believe that you can really heal from emotional trauma.

- *Have you been prescribed any medications to help you deal with the problems stemming from your trauma? What are the medications, and how effective have they been, both in addressing the short-term symptoms as well as in helping you to heal and lead a fulfilling, successful life?*

If you have tried medications, I hope that they helped at least somewhat. Zoloft, Prozac, Wellbutrin, Abilify, Seroquel, Effexor, Trazodone, Ambien, and others are all typically prescribed for a diagnosis of PTSD. Again, I think medications can assist in trauma treatment, but as you may have experienced, medications may work, but only until you stop taking them, either because you don't like the side effects, hate being dependent on them, or even become frustrated with the whole process. Medications may help with some trauma symptoms, but as soon as you stop the medications, your symptoms will return. As previously referenced,[3] most medications will help some, however, without the addition of effective psychotherapy, all medications are prone to a relapse in symptomology when the medication is stopped.

- *How much work on your issues have you done on your own? Did your therapist suggest you should be working on healing outside of his/her office? Did your therapist give you any tools or techniques to use on your own?*

If you have attempted to work on these issues on your own, kudos to you, because that requires a great deal of courage. The odds are, though, that your therapist didn't encourage this or didn't provide you with tools and techniques to do so. Healing can be done at home, and I will often recommend that people use various techniques such as cognitive exercises or writing letters to help themselves when they are not in session. While the typical Cognitive Behavior (CBT) therapist will assign you homework to complete (e.g., thought records, behavioral interventions, and various worksheets), remember that it's not simply the amount of time you spend on healing, but *how you spend the time.* Working to heal through remembering, feeling, expressing, releasing, and reframing are critical, active techniques, and so using these techniques is far more important than spending huge amount of times doing less critical activities.

- *How has the emotional trauma you suffered affected your life negatively? Has it negatively affected you in terms of careers, relationships, moods, or your ability to enjoy life? Has therapy helped you deal successfully with any of these problems, especially in the long-term?*

There are subtle ways and then there are obvious ways that experiencing trauma can impact one's life. Working too much, as Jim did, is an example of an obvious response to his trauma. More subtly, he lost his enjoyment of life because his mind was anchored in the past. **Therapeutic treatment is designed to address and permanently resolve these issues. Anything less is ineffective treatment.**

Many people are dissatisfied with their emotional trauma treatment; and people who have stopped treatment or never bothered with it may grit their teeth and try to muddle through life with all the burdens that trauma creates.

It doesn't have to be this way. To help make the case for an effective alternative and a model for trauma treatment, let me share six different approaches that have contributed to my model on healing from emotional trauma. In this way, I think you'll start to understand the roots of trauma and how it might respond to the right treatment protocols.

SIX CONTRIBUTIONS TO MY UNDERSTANDING AND TREATMENT OF EMOTIONAL TRAUMA

Before introducing my model for treating trauma, let's explore trauma from six distinct perspectives: those of stress response, neuroscience, cognitive behavioral theory, Gestalt Theory, Freudian psychoanalysis, and religious training. Each of these topics will provide insight into the method I use and why it is so effective in the treatment of all types of emotional trauma.

The Stress Response

In 1956, Dr. Hans Selye at the University of Montreal described in his book a three-step response to challenges, which he called the stress response[5]. More specifically, he coined the term General Adaptation Syndrome[6] (GAS) to illustrate a three-step progression of what happens to an organism (including you, the human) when stressed. Selye noted that stress is a specific, predictable, internal response to a non-specific stimulus or threat. In other words, whatever threatens you, be it a subpoena, an IRS audit, or an episode of Real Housewives of New Jersey, evokes a predictable physiological response: secretion of stress hormones like norepinephrine and cortisol, accelerated heart rate and respiration, shutdown of digestion and sexuality, and increased blood flow to the major muscle groups, including the chest, back, arms, and legs, all of which prepares the organism for "fight or flight."

This first stage is called the alarm reaction, and it is entirely normal and appropriate. The extra fuel you receive from norepinephrine, for instance, aids you in staying up all night for the final exam or rescuing a child from a burning house. When the threat is over, the body returns to homeostasis.

The second stage of the GAS is the "resistance stage." Here, the stressor is ongoing, so your nervous system remains in high gear. For example, your high-conflict marriage becomes a high-conflict divorce, your financial woes worsen, or your child's hyperactivity continues unabated. This stage lasts as the perceived stressor goes on—or until the body's coping mechanisms give way to the third stage, "exhaustion."

Exhaustion is exactly what you think it is, a breakdown of the nervous system resulting in fatigue, dysphoria (low mood), anhedonia (an inability to experience pleasure from previously rewarding activities), free-floating anxiety, insulin spikes, panic attacks, infections of all kinds (since your immune system no longer fights off intruders), muscle cramping and aching, every one of your least favorite gastrointestinal symptoms, and so much more. People in the third stage are hospitalized or suffer from "nervous breakdowns," depressive episodes, psychotic breaks, or panic attacks. Our coping mechanisms are temporarily defeated and require help.

So what does this have to do with treatment of trauma? Unresolved trauma causes the stress response to be left in the "on" position, or perhaps it is like a faucet that is continually running. A primary goal of treatment is to shut off the stress response, return it to the "off" position, or shut off the faucet, whatever analogy you prefer.

And how is that done? The mind must believe that there is no longer a threat (or that it is manageable) and that all is "okay." It's that simple. And yet meeting this condition is imperative for turning off the stress response. In reality, there are a thousand ways to get to "okay." For instance, the surgeon looks down at you in the recovery room, smiles, and says, "We got it all, you will recover completely," and you believe her. Likewise, the insurance guy calls and says, "We've reviewed your case, and we are going to pay for 100 percent of the flood damage," and you believe him. Your wife says the affair is over and she only wants to be with you, and you believe her. The nanny says she will forgive your children for tying her up in the playroom and will not resign after all, and you believe her.

Again, the mind must conclude that somehow all is okay once again for the stress response to be shut down. So you, the trauma sufferer, need to believe that whatever the trauma—rape, betrayal, financial loss, death of a loved one, abandonment, the sounds and images that form the experience of combat, etc.—there is hope, and you and it will be okay. For Jim to resolve his issue, he will have to believe that despite the loss of his two sons, he can recover and live a meaningful life. All will be okay.

Neuroscience

Trauma can quite literally change your brain[7]. Various neurological studies and research conducted since Selye's discovery of the stress response have further illuminated the impact that trauma can have on brain structure.[8][9] Thanks to modern neuroimaging, we can now observe some of the fascinating complexities of the brain. For instance, the hippocampus is the structure responsible for memory. More specifically, it creates new memories, storing them away for later, and also retrieves memories in the brain. If I ask you to recall the name of your third-grade teacher, more than likely, you would be calling upon your hippocampus to do the dirty work. But as Bremner (2006) notes, it appears trauma is responsible for reducing the volume or size of the hippocampus.[7]

Why does size matter? Since we routinely call upon our memory center thousands of times in the course of a day, shrinkage would create confusion and compromise your capacity for recall. Additionally, a smaller hippocampal unit would make it more difficult to decipher which things were threatening to you and which not. Your judgment would also be reduced, and the stress response would be triggered far too often by non-threatening stimuli.

After a particularly bad auto accident, the hippocampus may be impacted. As such, deciphering what driving conditions are normal and which ones are dangerous may be extremely difficult. Hence, all driving on crowded roads and highways might be perceived as very threatening and compromise the driver's willingness or confidence in his/her ability to drive. Again, this may contribute to your stress response being left in the "on" position for no good reason.

The limbic system, the area of the brain most responsible for emotions, contains the amygdala, which is thought to be responsible for emotional processing and the acquisition of fear responses. Your amygdala attempts to determine what a given stimulus is and whether or not to react emotionally to the stimulus. When adversely impacted by trauma, this structure in the brain is thought to become "hyper-responsive" in trauma clients. This means that not only does your brain react too strongly to trauma, but also to ANY emotional stimuli; this overreaction can be measured in cortisol levels in your blood plasma and saliva.[10][11] You might find yourself crying uncontrollably during a sad part in a movie, or overreacting in fear to a bathroom spider with a handlebar mustache. This would mean that your emotional reactions to items NOT associated with the trauma would be far greater than would otherwise be anticipated. You can imagine how exhausting life would be if everything felt frightening and required you to be on high alert. This is the experience of many combat veterans, including those I have known who have kept watch throughout the night, checking and rechecking the locks on the door and the safety of their children.

As you may know, the brain is divided into four lobes: frontal, parietal, temporal, and occipital. The frontal lobe is responsible for things like personality, decision-making, initiation of activity, emotional reactivity (how one responds to emotions), motivation, social interactions, and even judgment. Evolutionarily speaking, this is the last part of your brain to develop, and it does not stop growing until your early twenties. It is this very same frontal lobe that scientists claim separates us as humans from all other creatures on the planet.

Any trauma that occurs can impact your brain functioning. Within the frontal lobe is the medial prefrontal cortex (mPFC). The mPFC is responsible for inhibiting the stress response, which is housed in the amygdala. Koenigs and Grafman (2009) noted that people exposed to trauma had a decreased activity volume in their frontal cortex, more specifically in the mPFC.[12] Why is this decreased activity important to PTSD? If the area of the brain responsible for shutting off the stress response is left on, the stress response continues. Continued stress can then lead to more unhealthy responses to difficult and stressful situations, including drinking alcohol to excess, angry responses, and even social isolation.

The bottom line is this: trauma impacts the structures of the brain, making life considerably more difficult for the survivor. Healing from the traumatic event(s) becomes that much more necessary.

Consider how Jim's brain may have responded to his trauma. With traumatic impairment of his hippocampus, he reportedly perceived two young boys in the barbershop as too closely resembling his deceased boys, which therefore launched his body into a full-blown panic attack. His under-responsive prefrontal cortex (PFC) didn't properly regulate his over-reactive amygdala and may have made normal challenges during his work at the auto shop feel overwhelming to him. Fortunately, these changes in the brain can be addressed with good treatment and healing.

COGNITIVE BEHAVIORAL THERAPY

Cognitive Behavioral Therapy, usually just called CBT, was developed by Albert Ellis in the 1960s and Aaron Beck in the 1970s.[13] CBT holds that our thoughts and beliefs influence how we behave and feel. Such beliefs include how we view ourselves, how we view others, and how we view the world. One person sees himself as inferior, while another sees himself as superior. You perceive your mother as supportive, your sister sees her as critical. One person sees the world as warm and welcoming, the other sees the world as cold and harsh. And as your therapist will tell you is true, how you perceive something is more important than reality when it comes to your feelings and emotions. Said simply, when it comes to your emotions, perception trumps reality (and that is not a political statement).

How Beliefs about Self, Others, and the World Are Developed

Self-views relate heavily to concepts like self-esteem, self-worth, and self-confidence. All of this supports a concept that psychologists call "self-efficacy."[14] When good things happen, it is either because "I worked for it" or because "I got lucky." Views of self are influenced heavily by parental praise and punishment. Were your parents highly critical of you? If so, then you may think, "I'm not good enough," and that "No one will ever love me." On the other hand, if your parents affirmed not only your success, but also your efforts, you may "try and try again."

Views of others play out heavily in relationships. Was your trust betrayed by someone important to you? Maybe your father said he would show up at your baseball games, but never did. When the people you love let you down, trust becomes an issue.

Views of the world come into play in the work environment, in the community, in government, and for the world as a whole. Is work a competitive place where coworkers backstab each other for promotions? Or is it a place where people cooperate to get the job done? What about government? Are politicians motivated to do good, or are they inherently corrupt?

Cognitive Beliefs or Schemas

The cognitive perspective on human behavior is especially important in explaining how pathological behavior endures over time. Beck (2011) explained that in psychology, views of self, others, and the world go by a technical name; they are called cognitive beliefs or schemas.[13] Your beliefs provide a readymade mold into which your experiences are poured. We've all had the experience of responding in a knee-jerk fashion, in a rush to judgment that seems to ignore objective facts. This happens because your beliefs influence other interpretations of experience. People *tend to* fall back on pre-existing biases and prejudices (the beliefs one brings to the experience). We have to. The world is far too complex, and our cognitive abilities are far too limited, for our perspectives on life to be invented anew with each rising sun. Instead, we apply what we have been taught, usually by parents, role models, education, and other previous experiences in life. We have beliefs about ourselves, others, the world, and the future. These beliefs are usually accepted as facts because we just don't have time to isolate and test the assumptions that underlie all of our thoughts and actions. From our belief system, certain thoughts, feelings, and behaviors arise. As an example, if you believe you are unworthy and unlovable, a friend cancelling their plans to hang out with you might invoke feelings of rejection, while at the same time your friend might have a very good reason why they had to cancel their plans.

Cognitive Therapy and PTSD

This is especially true with PTSD, where the very structure of memory and cognition are changed by a traumatic event. When clients tell me they "can't remember what happened," they are really saying that their physiological arousal at the time of the traumatic event was so intense that they cannot recall the details of their experience. This is called "state-dependent memory,"[15] which means simply that the state of the body is encoded along with the objective facts of the experience. When the state of your body changes, your memory may not be easily accessible. Symptoms of numbing dampen emotions and prevent traumatic material from reaching your conscious awareness. Hypervigilance (being overly watchful) supports a sense of safety by ensuring that the individual attends to every possible threat. At the same time, it ensures that you perceive threats that don't really exist, mobilizing your fight-or-flight system to deal with each such "emergency," even if the loud noise was only thunder, and not enemy mortars.

Because PTSD changes the very architecture of cognition, it is necessary for your therapist to interpret your statements liberally. Your reluctance to cooperate in therapy can mean either, "I don't think I'm strong enough to say this out loud," or "Talking about the traumatic event makes it real again." When you say, "I can't move on," you may be referring to flashbacks or intrusive memories that suddenly return to your mind. Or alternatively, you may be saying, "I can't move on due to guilt... What happened was my fault." The term "survivor's guilt" refers specifically to this phenomenon. Survivor's guilt occurs sometimes when you survive a traumatic event where others died.[16] "I should've died along with my mother, father, brother, sister, child, or fellow soldiers." Survivor's guilt may lead to "self-flagellation," that is, punishing yourself for "letting loved ones die on my watch." This includes any behavior with a high potential for painful consequences, such as risk-taking (e.g., excessive speeding), self-harming (e.g., cutting), self-neglect (e.g., drinking, drugs, loss of jobs and relationships), and not seeking treatment (in order to continue the misery of unresolved trauma). Careful inspection shows that self-blame is actually based on the expectation or assumption that life should be fair for everyone. Life is not fair, and the consequences can be tragic, particularly when you attempt to take responsibility for events beyond your control.

For Jim, schemas (or beliefs about self, others, and the world) about himself became more and more prominent as therapy progressed. "I'm the worst father ever," he confessed. Not a single day passed in Jim's life that he didn't feel guilty for what happened to his sons. If you tell yourself the same thing every day for forty-five years, you are likely to believe it. Jim perceived himself as a failure. Not only did he fail to find his sons when he drove into the water, he was still alive. "If only it could have been me," he thought. "Why couldn't it have been me? Why didn't I check the ice? Why am I still alive when my boys are dead?" Taking responsibility for the impossible was Jim's way of remaining connected to his sons, his attempt to turn a wish into reality. As long as Jim believed that he was "the worst father ever," he deserved whatever misery he could bring on himself. To be whole again, Jim needed to let go, and **he needed to realize that letting go was not an abandonment of his sons.**

Before I go any further, I would like to state that there is a lot of research conducted on the effectiveness of CBT for PTSD treatment. Research has shown repeatedly that CBT is indeed effective in the treatment of PTSD. In a particularly good research study done by Nilamadhab Kar (2011), a meta-analysis conducted using thirty-one randomized control studies, the "gold standard" of psychological research, showed that CBT had successfully reduced trauma-related symptoms in people who were victims of terrorism, combat, sexual assault, refugees, and motor vehicle accidents, as well as disaster survivors.[17] So far, so good, right? Another meta-analysis of fifty-five studies of empirically supported treatments for PTSD found that nonresponse and dropout rates were as high as 50 percent.[18] This meant even odds, or the flip of a coin on whether or not you'd get better or drop out of treatment, or not very good chances, to my mind, and as I'll explain later, I think there is a reason for this. Yet CBT is still a major contributor to my theory on how you can heal from trauma.

FREUDIAN THEORY

I've never been a Freudian, not even a little bit. I never liked his theories on psychosexual development and especially disliked his (over)emphasis on sex, aggression, and the unconscious. But admittedly, I have been profoundly influenced by Freud in two ways, especially as it relates to my theory on healing from a pain in the past.

First, I think Freud's writings on defense mechanisms were pure genius. The defenses he described are still widely accepted today by most practitioners

...ful and spot-on, including denial, minimization,
...ent.[19] But when it comes to treating trauma
...sm that stands out above the others to
...ocumented that horrific trauma can be so
...only possible mode of survival is to block even
...experience from the delicate mind. It really happened,
...d in the brain (in complete detail and living color for future
...but for now, there is a free pass to survive without the ugly movie
...your head. The mind, it appears, is attempting to block the images, the
way your mom put her hands over your eyes during the naughty parts of the
movie. The memory is frozen, presumably in your hippocampus, only to be
triggered some time in the future by an otherwise benign event. Whatever
was frozen is now defrosted and fresh, as if it had just happened. Good
therapy requires that it (finally) be dealt with and put away successfully in
order to return the stress switch back to the "off" position.

Similarly, Freud postulated that the goal of good therapy (psychoanalysis)
was to make the unconscious conscious.[20] In other words, in order to heal,
the trauma must be processed on a conscious level. Hence, the material
that has never been allowed to surface (and is thus neither remembered,
felt, nor expressed) cannot be released to allow the client to heal. From all
indications, Freud, it turns out, was exactly right. That is, no healing will
occur until you consciously process and release your traumatic memory.

GESTALT THERAPY

The great German theorist and psychologist Fritz Perls is one of the most
underrated and underappreciated contributors to modern psychology and
especially to psychotherapy. If I asked twenty recent doctoral residents
in psychology the question of who are the top five greatest contributors

to their style of practice, I don't know if I I'd hear the name mentioned even once.

So why do I deem him to be so influential and necessary in such recovery from trauma? His Gestalt (the German word for the whole picture, entity, or enchilada) theory emphasizes closure, or completion of unfinished business.[21] Who do you know that mows 90 percent of their lawn? Makes half the bed? Shaves one leg? We have a need to complete things, to put things away or find a better place for them psychologically. It's a phenomenon I observe every day in my office. Someone presents feeling stressed and overwhelmed because of their perception of a given situation in their lives. By the end of the session they feel dramatically relieved and better—not because the world has changed, but because they perceive an opportunity to place something painful, scary, or threatening in a better place where it loses its power to upset them. With unresolved trauma, clients cannot seem to let go of their horror because it is unfinished for them. Whether it is blocked partially or completely from their memory (repression), repeats endlessly on a loop, or recurs every night in a nightmarish dream, it is only because it is unfinished.

Jim needed to "finish" his trauma by saying goodbye to his sons and forgiving himself for his perception of his having allowed them to die. He also needed to forgive God[22] for "taking his sons away from him." Finally, he had to believe that he had a life where he could find happiness.

RELIGION AND FORGIVENESS

Pick a religion, any religion. With the exception of perhaps Satanism, virtually all religion teaches the necessity of forgiveness for living a godly life and achieving peace, wholeness, and connection with the divine. In Buddhism, forgiveness is about removing unhealthy emotions that would otherwise cause harm to the non-forgiving person. Likewise, Sikhism describes forgiveness as the remedy to anger, especially when the forgiving person is aroused by compassion. Judaism requires forgiveness after a sincere apology, but even in its absence, forgiveness is considered a pious act. Islam is a term derived from a Semitic word meaning peace. Forgiveness is thought to be a prerequisite for achieving peace.[23]

In Christianity, Jesus taught his followers to pray to God the father, "Forgive us our debts, as we forgive our debtors" (Matthew 6:12, King James Version). Note that he already assumes that we ought to be forgiving others, as it is essential to improve our own status with God. Jesus went on to say, "but if ye forgive not men their trespasses, neither will your Father forgive your trespasses." (Matthew 6:15, King James Version.)

Perhaps it is fair to conclude that forgiveness is that which lets the afflicted off the hook, as much or more than the offender. How is that so? Because the opposite of forgiveness, resentment or hatred, is known to be a toxin for the grudge holder. A twentieth-century Buddha, Mark Twain, quipped, "Anger is an acid that can do more harm to the vessel in which it is stored them to anything on which it is poured."[24] Research has confirmed that resentment contributes to numerous conditions, including depression, heart disease, and premature death.[25]

But what exactly is forgiveness? Let's begin with what it isn't. Psychologist Syd Simon taught that forgiveness is not forgetting; it is not revenge, nor does it condone the offense. Forgiveness, in the simplest sense of the word, means to let go.[26]

This translates into two types of forgiveness: forgiveness without reconciliation and forgiveness with reconciliation. They both allow for letting go of the offense, but one restores the relationship to the place or position held prior to the perceived offense, while the other does not. (Think of this as

"Mounds Bar" and "Almond Joy;" they are both the same candy, but one has nuts, and the other doesn't.)

For example, I once employed an office manager who admitted to embezzling funds from the practice. She was terminated on the spot. Several weeks later, I was completely over any hurt, anger, resentment, and sense of betrayal. But I did not rehire her. I forgave, but without reconciliation.

This is as opposed to the couples I've counseled after one of them committed infidelity and/or other egregious offenses. To aim for a happy marriage— or life—there must be forgiveness (letting go) with reconciliation. In that context, forgiveness must be repeated thousands of times in a fifty-year marriage, hopefully for lesser violations. Recall the Jesus quote when asked by Peter, "Lord, how oft shall my brother sin against me, and I forgive him? Till seven times?"

Jesus answered, "I say not unto thee, until seven times: but until seventy times seven," or indefinitely (Matthew 18:22, King James Version).

When working with trauma clients, my chief goal is to help them live in the present, while looking forward to the future. Consider whether this is a goal you've achieved. You should be able to remember the past, laugh, and tell stories about painful events and the lessons learned from them. But you should not be stuck in the past with pain, avoidance, resentment, intrusive recollections, recurrent nightmares, or excessive guilt, etc. These symptoms point to unresolved pain in the past and require forgiveness, or letting go.

MODERN DAY PROPHET?

An eighty-two-year-old woman sat on my couch one day and said, "So what I'm hearing you say, doctor, is that you want me to let go of everything that makes my head crazy." She was no prophet, but to me, that remains the best definition of forgiveness I've ever heard. In the chapters ahead, I will show you how you can learn to let go of those things that make your head crazy. Remember that by definition, what you don't let go of, you hold onto for the rest of your life. More importantly, the unresolved trauma owns you for the rest of your life.

What counterbalances the horrible stories that trauma clients tell me is their ability to finish their traumas once and for all. In the chapters to come, I will refer back to these six contributors and describe how their emphasis on closure and release comes to life in my approach to overcoming trauma. In fact, I've named the procedure after Fritz Perls, as a tribute to his brilliant understanding of healing from pain in the past. In chapter three, I'll explain what "The Fritz" entails and how you can apply it to your unfinished business.

Questions for Comprehension

—

What are the three best ideas that you gleaned from this chapter?

_____

_____

_____

_____

_____

What type of action do you believe is necessary to help actualize these ideas?

_____

_____

_____

_____

_____

How did you execute your plan?

_____

_____

_____

_____

_____

What is the result of your efforts?

_____

_____

_____

_____

_____

Chapter Two

Trauma Destroys the Soul Thanks to Mr. Avoidance

"Now, don't hang on. Nothing lasts forever but the Earth and sky. It slips away, and all your money won't another minute buy. Dust in the wind, all we are is dust in the wind. Everything is dust in the wind."
—Kansas

TRAUMA IS BAD

◇

You know about the nightmares, the insomnia, the rage, and the deep despair and hopelessness. The hypervigilance (constantly watching and scanning) makes you feel crazy, and the exaggerated startle response (jumping when unexpectedly tapped on the shoulder) is downright embarrassing. Your anxiety remains high, and your intrusive recollections of the event are just that, intrusive. They ruin your conversations, your productivity, your peace of mind. You look at the world through a glass darkly, as if someone had blotted out the sun permanently. You may still smile, but not as frequently or as sincerely. You can't remember when you were last at peace.

But trauma has many effects, many of which aren't widely known.. For instance, we now know that trauma is a big contributor to substance abuse. Research studies have noted repeatedly that traumatic experiences are associated with an increased risk of substance abuse. Najavits, Weiss, and Shaw (1997) noted that of women who experienced childhood physical or sexual assault, between 30–59 percent go on to develop substance abuse problems.[28] Another study found that out of thirty-eight male veterans who were placed in an inpatient substance abuse clinic, 77 percent of them had been exposed to severe childhood abuse.[29] Another study shows, again, that the prevalence of PTSD among chemically dependent adolescents is five times that of their peers who are free of such dependency.[30]

There's more; recent research from Newtown, Connecticut, after the school shootings suggest that when experienced by children, traumatic events are tremendous contributors to many symptoms and illnesses, especially mental illness and addiction behaviors. When children had gone through six or more traumatic events between birth and age eighteen (defined as an incident of physical or sexual abuse, parental arrest, or parental conflict, etc.), children had a 4,600 percent greater chance of using recreational intravenous drugs than those who had none.[31]

Katelyn was an IV drug user who preferred shooting crystal meth as her drug of choice. It took me several inpatient hospital visits to learn that she had been a victim of human trafficking in her teens and had been forced into prostitution. She was physically and sexually assaulted repeatedly, totaling "about 20" traumatic incidents. Little wonder, then, that she found solace in mood-altering chemicals.

Trauma is also linked with mental illness. You know about PTSD, depression, anxiety, and now addictions. Trauma is also a contributor to psychotic illnesses and is the cornerstone of dissociative illnesses, especially Multiple Personality Disorder (now called Dissociative Identity Disorder) and possibly also of Bipolar Disorder. A client of mine who had been diagnosed with Bipolar Disorder as a teen once said candidly to me, "I was never bipolar before I was abused."

Dr. Steven Sharfstein, former President of the American Psychiatric Association (APA), has said, "Smoking is to cancer as trauma is to mental illness."[32] Let me summarize with one of my own quotes, "Unresolved trauma is bad."

TRAUMA SYMPTOMS
ARE UNDERSTANDABLE

If you accidentally hammered your thumb (to the delight of the nail), several predictable responses would occur within the afflicted area: your thumb would throb, swell, and likely turn the color of a California plum, all because of the body's natural inclination to heal itself.

The mind is very much a part of the same system and also responds in a predictable manner. All trauma symptoms, as painful and dysfunctional as they may appear, are rooted in survival. While some of them may seem incomprehensible to the untrained eye, they all make sense when viewed within this survival context.

This context will become apparent as you read further, but here, let's use an analogy that helps illustrate how PTSD symptoms function: the splinter in my middle toe.

One afternoon at the office, my client failed to show up for an appointment, so I had a free hour to myself. The top of the middle toe on my right foot had been sore to the touch for several months, so I decided to remove my shoe and sock to investigate. The top of the toe was layered with excess skin, unlike any of the other toes. Looking below the skin, I saw a black dot embedded deeply in the toe. I decided to scratch at the layers of skin to remove the excess from the toe in order to gain access to the black dot. I squeezed the toe, only to reveal a small amount of liquid pus encasing a half-inch long wood splinter. Upon removal of the splinter, the excess skin did not grow back, and the toe never hurt again.

And then it occurred to me—my middle toe story is a perfect metaphor for Post-Traumatic Stress Disorder. Let's explore the metaphor further. My toe, unbeknownst to me, was traumatized by a very intrusive splinter. The splinter was invasive and did not belong within the toe; it needed to be expelled. But the owner/operator of the toe was oblivious to the intruder and only remotely connected to the pain. As such, the intrusive splinter remained. Since the splinter was not being removed, the body found it necessary to protect the toe from further attacks and sensitivity to the pain by providing the protective coating of excess skin. In this way, the toe (and the surrounding foot) was still quite functional despite the now buried and well-protected splinter. And yet, because something was wrong, pain and discomfort were the result.

Your system is designed for survival and will do what is necessary to keep you, the traumatized organism, alive at all costs. In the case of the toe, the protection was most important, even more important than removing the splinter. The layers of excess skin were evidently designed to allow the foot to continue to function despite the intruder. If cells of the toe could communicate, they might say, "This splinter has invaded our world and needs to be removed. But until that happens, our job is to protect the toe and keep the foot functional."

But the toe *was* communicating pain, which we understand is the body's way of relating that something is wrong. The message of consistent pain for several months should have been a good enough signal to me that there was something wrong. Only when I finally addressed the pain and removed the splinter did the toe return to normal.

And from my extensive work with trauma survivors, that is exactly how it works. When the traumatic episode(s) is satisfactorily digested (removed, assimilated, and released), the need for the PTSD symptoms fades away.

SURVIVAL MECHANISMS SEND CONFLICTING MESSAGES

But sometimes the PTSD symptoms send very conflicting messages: you need to remove the splinter (trauma), but I will try to bury it so you won't or don't have to deal with it. The repeatedly molested child, for instance, is often incapable of addressing her traumatic experiences while she's still young. Consequently, the mind's protective system may allow her to block the ugly traumas out for many years to promote her survival until she is finally equipped to deal with her abuse, often many years later.

Contradictory messages from your protective mindset serve a purpose. A middle-aged Terri tells me the story of surviving a "home invasion," where the intruder grabbed wallets, cash, and jewelry before stumbling down the stairs and escaping into the night. She presents one month later with the predictable PTSD symptoms; she continues to re-experience the event, especially running after him and yelling "who are you?," and then watching him fall and run away. The nightmares and flashbacks do very much the same thing—remind her that her trauma (like the splinter) has not yet been dealt with.

There are symptoms of avoidance: buying an alarm system and not wanting to sleep alone (she invites her eleven-year-old to snuggle with her as they're both "spooked" by the violation). She also checks and re-checks locks as if they weren't successfully locked the last three times she locked them. And of course, she is experiencing the exaggerated startle response, hypervigilance, and excessive anxiety. This is all easy to understand, since Terri no longer perceives her world as safe since the home invasion.

From one perspective, Terri's symptoms are functional. She needs to successfully process the trauma to release it, so flashbacks and intrusive recollections are useful. The avoidance symptoms of feeling a need to buy a house alarm and check locks (not to an excessive OCD level) are logical responses to the home invasion. Even the startle response and hypervigilance are ingrained reflexes designed to keep Terri alive and well.

From another perspective, though, Terri's symptoms are irrational. Let's say you're a driver returning to the road after an automobile accident. Your goal should not be hypervigilance, only appropriate caution. You don't need to check your side mirrors twenty-seven times, two should suffice. Alert is good, but employing the "grip of terror" upon the steering wheel is not.

For Terri, being hyper-aroused (extreme anxiety) and watching for potential intruders and assorted bad guys seems appropriate, but more than likely, it will do more harm (in terms of insomnia, anxiety, and depression, as well as irritability, family conflict, and poor work performance) than good. Again, appropriate vigilance, checking the doors and having a dog and/ or a non-canine alarm system makes sense. Hypervigilance, not so much.

Terri grasps how her symptoms have crossed the line. But letting go of these symptoms—putting them away—is a challenge because her mind's protective system may fight to retain them due to their perceived usefulness. In other words, letting go of the checking, the worrying, the relentless scanning, and her overreaction to the shadow created by her standup Hoover vacuum may make Terri feel vulnerable. She may resist giving up her newfound internal security system.

So, what can be done to help Terri to let go of her disruptive PTSD symptoms while retaining a healthy—not careless, not excessively guarded—system of self-protection? Let's talk treatment.

TRAUMA (PTSD) IS TREATABLE

Needless to say, if trauma were not treatable (and yes, very often curable), there would be no reason to write this book. But there is successful treatment, and it's about time someone taught it to you. Now that you understand how trauma symptoms are at least in part functional and are built to sustain or preserve life, you possess a perspective that will facilitate treatment—a perspective on how to use the Fritz.

Fritz Perls, as you remember from Chapter 1, was the German-born psychotherapist who founded the Gestalt school of therapy. Perls and Gestalt therapy were tremendously popular in the '50s and '60s, but Perls' work at the Esalen Institute in Big Sur alienated traditional therapists who didn't like how some people were embracing it as a lifestyle (i.e. mindfulness, meditation, etc.). Over time, some of Gestalt's general concepts were absorbed into the Cognitive-Behavioral school, but many of Perls' brilliant innovations were lost after his death in 1970.

Perls emphasized closure.[33] He believed, as do I, that the issues with which humans struggle have power over us—think the stress response—until we find a way to close the wound. Again, that means putting these issues in a place where you can accept the trauma, both that it happened and that it cannot be changed, fixed, or undone. All you can do is accept it and then, perhaps, find meaning in your suffering and possibly create a plan to make your life better because of your resilience.

Recognize, though, that you have to go beyond a cognitive admission that the trauma occurred—that you were betrayed, abused, and so on—and that nothing can be done about it. For the splinter to be removed, you will need to face the pain from the trauma head-on, every aspect of it, and feel, express, and release the memories and the accompanying feelings before you can achieve acceptance, or make peace, shut off the stress response, remove the splinter, however you want to describe it. You must complete the horror of the trauma and the feelings you have been running from by expressing and releasing them. Dave's story illustrates this process nicely.

Years ago, the fire chief called me one day to discuss an emergency—twenty-six-year-old police trainee Dave had accidently been shot in the face with blanks during a training session. Sometime later, Dave's wife found him in the bathroom behind closed doors with a loaded gun in his mouth. He was now considering suicide because he couldn't deal with the recurrent nightmares of the shooting, night in and night out.

But why was the shooting returning to Dave on a nightly basis? Because he had not allowed himself to process and complete the trauma. The repetition of the event was the mind's way of alerting him that he was frightened and overwhelmed by the shooting and needed to express and release those feelings, once and for all.

Dave needed only one session of guided imagery (much more about this later in the book) to complete his trauma. Interestingly, he dreamed of his trauma one more time the night of our session and then never again. He had put the horror of the incident away for good.

Interestingly, in Dave's case, the severity of his symptoms, especially his suicidal thoughts, worked in his favor, because he was forced to get treatment and deal with the horror shortly after the trauma. Typically, police officers and other first responders are discouraged from thinking or talking about their traumatic experiences on the job, and they experience a disproportionately high rate of PTSD as a result.[34]

Putting on the Fritz

So here is the Fritz, a new paradigm for successful treatment of trauma/PTSD. It's a simple five-step process for treating PTSD. Fritz Perls, the German psychologist who inspired this process, would describe trauma and the associated symptoms as "unfinished business." He would remind the suffering client that the symptoms persist because they have not yet been completed and put in a healthier place. This simple idea—**that trauma will continue to dominate your mind, your body, and your life until you face it head on and release its hold over you**—is the very foundation of this treatment.

The steps are not necessarily as separate and distinct as they appear when written, but all are necessary to finish with your pain in the past and put away the symptoms. In real life, the steps will occur concurrently or blend into each other, and successful resolution of a trauma may occur in one session (as in Dave's case) or even by doing homework between sessions. With that introduction, here are the five steps:

> Remember: Tell the tale in detail.
> Feel: No feel, no heal.
> Express: Let the water flow.
> Release: Release for peace.
> Reframe: Reclaim your present life.

In my experiences, the steps of The Fritz work consistently, not occasionally, for trauma survivors who are brave enough to face their unfinished past pain. Later, I'll devote five chapters to explaining each of the five steps in depth. For now, though, keep these steps in mind as you read the stories of people who overcame their trauma to live great lives—and stories of those who did not.

The following story reveals the archenemy of the Fritz. While Batman has the Joker, and Luke Skywalker has Darth Vader, the Fritz has Mr. Avoidance.

Face the Past and Mr. Avoidance

The best way I can explain Mr. Avoidance is by telling the story of Orlando, a seventy-five-year-old man referred to me by his wife because of his fitful sleep pattern and terrible nightmares related to his time in military service. She had always been puzzled by Orlando's nocturnal suffering. He had been in the Navy but never saw combat. What could have happened to her husband?

Orlando was a proud man—he was a longstanding local legend in the twelve-step community, with over forty years of sobriety and a reputation for being a thorough but helpful sponsor. Despite his success in staying clean and sober and helping others to do the same, Orlando was miserable, and he was carrying a secret over fifty years old, dating back to his tenure in the Navy. He claimed that there was a story that he had never told anyone that had haunted him for years. Besides the sleep disturbance, he suffered from symptoms of depression and anxiety, in addition to a deep and pervasive shame of which evidently no one in the twelve-step community was aware. His prideful leadership was belied by the fact that he was still—fifty years down the road—a deeply wounded and conflicted man.

Orlando began telling me his story in the second session. It was why he was in treatment in the first place, to share his story and escape the weight of shame that was diminishing his life.

He told me that he was on a Navy ship when he was ordered below deck into the cramped private quarters of two of his superiors. He began to describe how the men ordered him as a young seaman to disrobe and prepare for what sounded like the beginning of an anal rape. Orlando paused for a moment and looked down at the floor, and when he finally looked up, he stood up and said, "I cannot do this. I'm sorry, I will not be back."

Orlando never returned to my office. I have questioned what went wrong; did I ask, "what happened" prematurely? I don't think so, but it's possible that I could have better prepared him for the feelings that he would experience when he told his story. The real blame, though, falls on the culprit that keeps so many trauma suffers silent—avoiding the horrible feelings that comprise the trauma. This avoidance keeps people like Orlando stuck in their pain in the past. Fortunately, Orlando is an exception, not the rule. The vast majority of clients I've worked with improved or were completely cured by their participation in treatment and their use of the Fritz. Orlando's story, though, serves as a cautionary tale about the dangers of how avoidance may prevent successful treatment.

Collateral Damage

While trauma contributes to depression, anxiety disorders, PTSD, dissociative disorders, and substance abuse, unresolved pain in the past can also contribute to a host of other symptoms and issues that can linger. For instance, trauma survivors often perceive the world as an unsafe place, feel isolated, withdraw emotionally from intimate relationships, can't trust others, tend to choose abusive relationships (to replicate the familiarity of an abusive childhood), and sabotage life's opportunities.

These symptoms don't automatically disappear after the original trauma has been successfully remembered, felt, expressed, and released. As the following story demonstrates, these symptoms can persist even after the original trauma has been faced and worked through.

Eighteen-year-old Kendra was in trouble for shoplifting—not what would be considered clinical grounds for a trauma diagnosis. Her dad, Tom, overheard her telling her long-distance boyfriend, "I don't know why these things keep happening to me—first I get molested by the babysitter, and now I'm arrested for shoplifting!" Imagine her dad's reaction when he overheard this conversation from the next room. Tom had never had an inkling that Kendra had been molested, and he didn't know what to do with the information.

He and his wife made an appointment to see me, but without Kendra. They arrived distraught and at a loss as to what to do. They explained that they had only used a babysitter once, and it was Tom's former best friend, Jim. Could that single occasion have been what Kendra was describing? And if so, what could they do about it now? I suggested that they return with Kendra and then tell her the truth about the overheard conversation, followed by the question, "Who was it that hurt you?"

They were shocked when Kendra confirmed that the culprit was indeed her dad's ex-best friend, during his one and only babysitting opportunity. Then I learned how much damage that one evening had done, including terrible shame, loss of innocence, and rebellion against everyone and everything (and yes, that's how a well-to-do girl who wants for nothing can find it permissible to shoplift).

There was even more damage that the entire family had sustained without ever realizing that it was caused by the abuse. According to Kendra, who was only nine at the time of the abuse, that was the day when she stopped trusting her parents—especially her dad—to protect her. It was dad's fault that Jim had touched her and then told her to tell no one. In her mind, dad had set her up for the abuse; and from her fourth-grade perspective, he was responsible for condoning, if not causing it. It was, after all, his best friend.

Further, that was also the day that Kendra had stopped being "daddy's little girl." That was the last time she had ever sat on his lap watching movies and eating popcorn, read aloud to him, or sought his advice on anything. He was not to be trusted for anything ever again.

So why hadn't her parents noticed the changes? Tom said he had noticed, and so had her mother, but ironically, they'd attributed her changes to growing up and needing less cuddles, less connections, less guidance—less dad. Sure, Tom missed her, but if she was growing up, he could accept her changes as a normal part of the growth process. After all, she was the first and only child, so what did he know about normal adolescent female development?

I suggested that Kendra work briefly with me to dispel the horror of the molestation. I used a technique called "Guided Imagery" that is used to complete the unfinished trauma and remove its hold over the survivor. I then asked Kendra how she felt. "Vanquished!" was her one-word reply (after all, she went to a school for the gifted).

But regardless of the success of the imagery, the damage to Kendra's relationship with her parents, especially her dad, was not magically repaired. She could release the horrors of the molestation, but that did not mean that all was automatically better with her parents. For that to happen, Kendra needed to hear their apologies, believe their innocence, and choose to trust them again.

Repairing a relationship can be a process, so Kendra gradually made the effort to be with her parents and talk, really talk, for the first time in nine years. During college, she took opportunities to return home and watch movies with her parents. She didn't sit on daddy's lap, but she was back to eating his popcorn and sitting between them.

Her symptoms waned and gradually disappeared. I've related Kendra's story because for at least some of you, it's not just the original trauma that's the problem, but a host of symptoms that originated with the trauma. The good news is that the Fritz can help you put away the trauma, and ongoing help specific to the collateral damage can also be immensely helpful in repairing the remaining damage. But for now, to help you capitalize on

the Fritz's healing power, let's look at the five steps in depth, starting
with Remembering.

Questions for Comprehension

—

What are the three best ideas that you gleaned from this chapter?

_____

_____

_____

_____

_____

What type of action do you believe is necessary to help actualize these ideas?

_____

_____

_____

_____

_____

How did you execute your plan?

_____

_____

_____

_____

What is the result of your efforts?

_____

_____

_____

_____

_____

Chapter Three

Remember: Tell the Tale in Detail

•

"It seems to me that there are more hearts broken in the world that can't be mended, left unattended. What do we do? What do we do?"

—Gilbert O'Sullivan

REMEMBER: TELL THE TALE IN DETAIL

Dennis was sixty-one years old when I met him. A delightful man with two somewhat inconsistent passions—NFL football and cross-dressing—he presented with some of the classic symptoms of depression, anxiety, and post-traumatic stress, all of which he believed had been caused by priest abuse, exactly fifty years ago.

Dennis was very discouraged; not only were his Dolphins in last place this season, but he believed he would never recover from his deep-rooted shame and self-contempt. Dennis had worked for the government consistently throughout his life but had always felt he was a failure. His interests could afford him temporary respite and escape from his sense of failure and disgust but never made him feel like a whole man or a worthwhile person or husband. Unfortunately, his wife could never understand why Dennis had so much self-contempt. She tolerated his cross-dressing, as she knew this was something that brought him a lot of excitement and positive feelings, though she didn't appreciate him spending more time in the bathroom on Saturday nights then she did.

In the second session I asked Dennis what had happened to him fifty years ago.

He said, "Do you mean with the priest?"

"Yes."

"You know, you are at least the fourth psychologist I've seen, and the first one to ask me what happened."

"What did you do with the others, exchange recipes?" I asked, demonstrating my amazement that in fifty years, he had never had to address the trauma, despite receiving professional help.

Dennis reluctantly began to share his stories of the sexual abuse, even though he felt emasculated by the tears and helplessness he experienced as he related the details of each episode. Dennis explained to me that he had never told anyone his story. After prompting him with the question of what had prevented him from doing so, he went on to tell me about the story of his brother. Dennis explained that one day, he and his little brother were in the back of one of the priest's cars driving to the church. There were two priests, one in the front seat with Dennis and one sitting with his brother in the back. Suddenly, his six-year-old brother blurted out, "Father Patrick is touching me!" The priest in the passenger seat turned his body all the way around and got in Dennis's brother face and yelled, "You will never speak of this again to anyone!" Dennis told me that he was in shock and speechless as both boys remained silent for the rest of the ride, gripped with fear. Three days later, in a terrible accident, Dennis' brother drowned in a pond near his house. Dennis believed that God himself had punished his brother for speaking against the priest, and that Dennis, in turn, was never to speak about what happened to him. He never did, until, of course, he and I began psychotherapy.

On approximately our sixth session, Dennis claimed, "Doc, this is just not working. It's getting worse. Now I am even dreaming about the priest. How is this supposed to help me if it's now infiltrating my dreams?"

I had a strong hunch that because he was relating his stories one by one, (this is the only way to successfully treat traumatic memories, one at a time,) he had stumbled upon another memory that was now manifesting itself in his dreams.

"Tell me about your dream."

"I don't know, I feel like he's coming into a room and whispering my name: Dennis, Dennis, where are you?"

Since it was already apparent to me that this was a memory couched in a dream, my job was simple: encourage him to complete the memory that was now surfacing.

"Where is this dream taking place?"

"Oh, s**t! I know where this is! We are away at a church weekend retreat. It's late at night, and all of us kids are asleep in a big room. Father Pat is creeping into the room trying to locate my bunk. I remember now—this is where it all started."

Dennis expressed his anguish, first in tears and then in some words of rage directed at the priest. I asked him to share everything he could remember about the incident until he had completely depleted his memory of these experiences.

Dennis never had this dream again. He didn't need to. He had processed the dream and the accompanying feelings, and he chose to release the ugliness of the rape in a letter directed to the priest (more on this technique in later chapters).

Dennis was in therapy with me for less than three months before he told me that for the first time in his life, he believed he was finally finished with the priest. (There were only three or four memories of being molested by him.) In fact, he claimed that the only time he ever thought about the priest abuse now was in my office, when I asked him about it. He sent me a Christmas postcard featuring strong words of affirmation for our work together on the back and a picture of himself in drag on the front.

It took Dennis time to remember in the right way, but time does not heal emotional wounds on its own. It merely passes. An entire half century had passed since he was molested by the priest. During that period, unfortunately, Dennis had only stewed silently because of the molestation. It is almost impossible for a child to separate from having experienced something ugly without the child feeling ugly herself or himself.

Dennis became the ugliness of the molestation. He lived nearly his entire life in shame and self-contempt. Only by having the opportunity to remember and process each of the memories could he finally reach a place of self-forgiveness and release the traumas.

THE MYTH THAT "TIME HEALS ALL WOUNDS"

The myth that time heals all wounds is pervasive in our society. In fact, it is even perpetuated by the mental health profession. How many psychotherapists are guilty of promising their clients that this (whatever it is) will get better over time? To those who believe that myth, I can introduce you to Vietnam veterans who are worse today than when they came home from combat in

1968. Similarly, I've met survivors of incest, rape, and family tragedies who have become more embittered over the years. Healing may occur over time, not because time passes, but because time affords you the opportunity to let go and make peace with the trauma.

It Is Letting Go, Not Time, That is the Ultimate Healer

The successful treatment of trauma requires the client to directly face the unresolved drama. This is known as exposure: one must remember the trauma in its entirety and deal with the accompanying feelings. But while exposure to painful material is necessary, it is not curative. The cure occurs because the client not only faces what happened (finally), but then feels, expresses, and most importantly, releases the painful emotions. In other words, exposure alone is the equivalent of only remembering the trauma and never processing it nor putting it away. It is the release of pain and fear that is ultimately curative.

Prolonged exposure is a technique that forces you to continue to re-experience the trauma. Ideally, you would habituate to the experience, meaning that it then no longer evokes that same magnitude of hurt or fear. In my experience, it is completely unnecessary to make anyone repeat the experience of trauma. To the contrary, one complete telling of the trauma, inclusive of the feelings (felt, expressed, and released), is sufficient to help you to make peace with your unresolved issue.

Remembering, of course, is only the first step of healing from your pain in the past. Trying to skip this step is as ill-advised as trying to skip first base on the way to second.

Linda and the Chicken Wire

Linda came to me many years ago with this simple request: "I just want to feel something. I am completely numb and feel absolutely nothing." At the time, I was unaware that Linda was blocking out the significant child abuse that had occurred when she was age four. She had been the victim of what is now called "human trafficking", as she was sold to various men in her community for sexual services while her single mother was working, and had entrusted her care to a great aunt and her boyfriend. As she began to remember some of the horrific incidents and the specific places and faces of the offenders, Linda became understandably upset. She did not want to continue with this process of healing from her terrible memories. In fact, she was in the process of remembering an incident where she was looking through chicken wire. Day after day and even in her dreams, she had a disturbing sense of being small and looking through holes in a chicken wire fence. Whatever that memory contained, Linda was not up for it. It was disturbing enough for her that she decided to take a break from treatment. That break lasted for five years before her depression intensified to the point that she decided she needed to finish what she had begun. During these five years, she remained stuck in a place of remembering looking through that chicken wire. When she returned to treatment, this was precisely the place to which we needed to return. She was finally capable of finishing remembering the story of being locked in a little crate from which she had looked out through chicken wire. By remembering and grieving through that terrible event, she never had another image, dream, or disturbing thought about the chicken wire again.

The healing process lasted for years—Linda had an unusually large number of abusive events to work through—until each one of her memories were remembered. But at the end of her treatment, two days after her final session, Linda called me to say she was experiencing feelings she had never had before and realized that these were feelings of happiness. She said it had taken her seventy years of life, and more than twenty years of therapy, to finally experience what it meant to be happy, but that had required flushing out all the ugliness of her childhood abuse.

Remembering rarely takes this long, but I relate Linda's case because it demonstrates how not remembering keeps people stuck. Despite doing her very best to run away from treatment, Linda could not escape the image of the chicken wire until she decided to face and process the memory. Only then did it go away forever, as it was finally finished.

EXPLORING MEMORIES

What if you can't trust the accuracy of your memories?

I know there are many of you who are skeptical as to whether the mind can repress memories for decades and then recall them in detail. While much debate has taken place on "recovered" versus "false" memories, it's not really an issue from a therapeutic standpoint. After more than thirty years of full-time practice and 70,000 therapy sessions, I have seen dozens of people who have repressed segments of (or entire) memories, all of whom were successfully treated when the memories were allowed to surface. The byproduct of a repressed memory surfacing has without exception been positive. Not one of my clients used the material to blame others for their lives; no one attempted to take anyone to court and sue them. The memories were ultimately digested and processed in such a way that they could now be integrated into the recovering person's life. I have read about people creating "false memories," but in my outpatient practice this has not been an obstacle to treatment.

Still, you may be skeptical: How do you know if you can completely trust the veracity of your memories? Generally speaking, we do not create false memories, as much as we confuse other data in our heads with what actually happened. For instance, Lenore Terr, a psychiatrist renowned for her work on repressed memories, wrote that based on her research, people do not make up a scene of being molested, for instance, but may confuse the color of the shirt the perpetrator was wearing with a different color that he had worn on another occasion.[36] Our memories may not be 100 percent factual, but they are crucial to recovery even if some details are not perfect.

Science has demonstrated that our memories are indeed fallible, which is a problem if you're trying to prove something in court. However, when it comes to treatment and recovery, perception, not fact, is king. It is perception, never reality, that creates emotion. Whatever you remember happened is what needs to be brought to the surface. Ultimately, the facts do not matter in this process; when it comes to healing, the emotions contained in the memory must be remembered, expressed, felt, and released.

I have spent hours with people remembering scenes from devil worshiping cults, wherein they describe horrible things from infanticide to daemonic or angelic presences. Did these things really happen? It is not up to me, the psychologist, to determine what from these memories is real. They are the memories and perceptions of the client. It is the expression and release of these memories that allows them to finish with the memory and complete their healing process. Remembering and working through their stories provides them with peace and healing about their respective childhoods. And remarkably, I have never needed to go back and redo a finished memory years later. What is finished remains finished for the rest of their lives. The healing takes place. While I make it a general practice to believe my clients, I don't ever need to validate their memories with anyone else, not with the perpetrators and not in a court room. Our work is strictly for the client's own benefit and never for forensic purposes.

What if you can't seem to remember?

I have worked with dozens of people who have been stuck, like Linda, in a kind of memory freeze-frame. Almost invariably, they can be gently prodded to unfreeze the memory and allow it to unspool. To create this memory movement, I typically ask them questions like "How old are you?" Where are you? What time of the day is it? Who is with you? What is happening? How do you feel?"

Jennifer came in with a great deal of discomfort about a repeating image in her mind. Her grandfather was chasing her around the dining room table when she was age six. I asked her how she felt at the time, hoping she would say amused and playful. Instead, she claimed that she was terrified that he would catch her. Through carefully worded questions, I helped her take me through a horrible summer of incest that she had suffered at his hands when her parents had left her with him while they were stationed overseas. Once she could deal with the first of these memories, the remainder of them followed suit, one at a time, until we were able to finish the stories and make peace with that entire chapter of her life.

Similarly, most clients are prepared to move past the stuck place when they present for treatment. Sometimes I ask them to do some relaxation and imagery or even self-hypnosis, but most of the time, they can access whatever is necessary to help them get unstuck and complete the healing.

But haven't you suffered enough? Isn't this treatment method cruel and unusual (punishment) treatment? Clearly you have suffered. The goal in treatment is to finish the horror show in your mind, not leave it stuck in an endless loop. For that to happen, you, the trauma sufferer, must finally address the horror by remembering it in totality, and then feeling, expressing, and releasing it.

Memory Avoidance

So if successful healing from trauma requires a visit to unfinished and undigested material, why do you, the survivor, avoid dealing with these memories as if they were a root canal? Only last week, while consulting with an eighty-year-old gentleman in the hospital with depression related to acute cardiac issues, I questioned him about his military service. He told me he had served in Vietnam, but added, "We don't talk about that."

But why not? Always remember that all behavior is purposeful and goal-oriented. You would not do something more than once unless you got something from it, and that includes avoidance. People avoid things that are uncomfortable to them. This is true from the first day of life (try blowing in the face of a newborn baby and watch the infant close her eyes and turn her head away). Similarly, take an elderly man on the last day of his life into a cold room and hear him request a sweater, a blanket, or a move to another room. You will frequently attempt to avoid discomfort, even when you might benefit from facing that discomfort.

To overcome the tendency of not remembering, keep the following four blockers in mind:

1. By holding on to your position of "victim," you can avoid all responsibility for being happy or successful. You always have the betrayal from your ex-husband or business partner or the physical abuse from your father on which to blame your unhappy life. To face the pain and finish it is tantamount to assuming responsibility for your own happiness and success. This can be very scary.

2. A traumatic memory or even painful losses can prompt you to erect a wall that will prevent you from ever being hurt again. Mary admitted that after her father died suddenly during her childhood, she has never allowed anyone to be that close to her. In all the relationships she's had, she has kept people at arm's length, especially by fault-

finding and emphasizing their negative attributes. To allow anyone to be intimately close to her would make her vulnerable to being hurt all over again, as when her father died.

3. Sometimes you believe if you should let go of the trauma or hurt, you would be condoning the perpetrator's bad behavior. I have had many people tell me that they will always hate their ex-husband for the affair and the subsequent abandonment, because to stop hating him would mean that he got away with his terrible behavior. Reviewing his "crime" on a regular basis feels like you are actively protesting that behavior. Forgiveness (letting go) would feel too much like accepting the bad behavior.

4. Facing the worst thing that ever happened to you is scary and painful, so you'd really prefer not to re-experience the terror and hurt. For this reason, you go to great lengths to avoid scary and painful issues, even if doing so guarantees that they will maintain their hold over you indefinitely. To deal with memory is to deal with frightening and painful emotion. And emotion, as you will see in the next chapter, is that which must be addressed and repaired for you to finally overcome your pain in the past.

How to Bring Back a Memory

Always remember that memories (including just regular, everyday memories) are fallible and imperfect re-creations of an actual event or events. Nonetheless, they can be incredibly accurate and informative, and they can be quite helpful to validate feelings you have held for many years. Very often, when the memories are traumatic, they have been repressed (blocked out of your conscious mind) for your protection. That does not mean they cannot be accessed, as very often they are stimulated many years later by current events. (Note the story of the traveling magician on page 78 under "Rick's Story.") While I am not an advocate of hunting for material to "prove" that someone has been abused or molested, people will present with fragments of a memory or at least an awareness that something has happened to them that they may have repressed. Sometimes they have a photograph in their head which is actually part of a repressed memory that is easy for them to stimulate in the safety of my office, but not at home.

As you'll see in the chapter on complex Post-Traumatic Stress Disorder, most multiple personality/Dissociative Identity Disorder (DID) clients will present with a very limited understanding as to what happened to them, who the different alter personalities are, or what they have to do to heal from past abuse. But once treatment begins, their memories are typically easily accessible.

If a memory is beginning to present itself, it is usually best to approach this in the safety of your mental health professional's office, especially if you're currently in therapy. It is okay to ask yourself how old you are, where you are, what time of day it is, whether you are alone or with others (who might be with you), and most importantly, what happens next? Little pieces will emerge, and it is important to allow yourself to see the movie that is now appearing in your head and to feel the accompanying feelings. It may be necessary to continue to ask yourself, "What happens next?" until the entire memory has surfaced. Typically, when the memory is completed and the feelings have been flushed out, the memory will stop presenting itself. Prior to that happening, the memory can be stuck in your head for weeks or longer, if it is not successfully extracted from its storage place (see the story of Linda and the "chicken wire" earlier in the chapter). Stories need to be told and felt and those emotions expressed and completely released in order to be completed.

Clients will often try to end their memory prematurely because they are frightened to find out what happens next, especially if they are about to be molested or raped or otherwise traumatized. Creating a different ending for a memory from the past is ill-advised, as it will not change what happened in reality. (This is another example of avoidance.) In my considerable experience, the memory will continue to torment the person until the truth is told in all its detail and that memory is completed. The memories that should be encouraged to surface are the ones that are already trying to force their way out by appearing in dreams, flashbacks, or intrusive recollections. Again, I would not go on a wild-goose chase looking for the potential of memories, but rather guide the client to finish whatever memory has already started to surface.

Without bringing out the memory, there will not be healing for a trauma survivor, and no integration will take place for a person with multiple personality disorder/DID. One of the most important items to consider when evaluating if a memory is finally over is whether there is finally a feeling of peace after the expression of the anxiety, pain, and tears. When memories are over, there is often a sense of peace that this has finally been expressed and released. If there is still anxiety present, that is typically an indication that there is more to the story that has yet to surface.

Finally, for the purposes of this section, you will know the memory is completed because it will no longer force its way to the conscious mind, since it is now satisfied. In cases where there are numerous memories, the next memory will begin to present itself shortly thereafter. Think of a Pez dispenser or a paper cup machine: when one is used, the next one will slide into position to be used next. (For a more complete understanding of this phenomenon, please see the chapter on complex Post-Traumatic Stress Disorder.) Finally, do not force the memory nor attach pieces to it that you are not certain happened. Be content to allow the memory to present itself until you feel quite certain that this is exactly what happened, even though you have temporarily blocked the memory to protect yourself from the horror of the feelings associated with the trauma.

If you are trying this at home, writing out the memory can be quite helpful. When writing a story, there is usually a beginning, a middle, and an end. Keeping this in mind will hopefully be quite helpful for you at home. Please feel free to write out whatever it is that you may have experienced as you read to the next sections.

Regarding where to start, there is no "right" answer. Very simply, if a memory is intact in your mind, start wherever it "makes sense" to begin. Again, think of a movie or a book; the beginning sets the stage for the rest of the story.

If you were a child when you were traumatized, ask yourself questions like:

- How old was I? Think of what grade you were in (first, third, elementary, middle school, etc.) might help anchor the time period.

- Where was I living at the time? If you moved at all, remember what house you were in, or what town or city.

- Who was in the house with me? Mom, dad, siblings, grandparents, etc.

- What was the quality of relationships you had with the people around you? They could have been good and close relationships, or perhaps Mom was typically angry, or Dad was never home, etc.

If you were in an abusive relationship or were sexually assaulted, ask yourself questions like:

- How did you two meet?

- Where did you two meet?

- What attracted you to him or her (if you were an adult at the time)?

- Were there any indications that something bad was going to happen?

If you are grief-stricken, ask yourself questions like:

- How old were you when the beloved one passed?

- What happened?

- What were the circumstances around what happened.

- What do you miss most about him/her?

Questions for Comprehension

—

What are the three best ideas that you gleaned from this chapter?

_____

_____

_____

_____

_____

What type of action do you believe is necessary to help actualize these ideas?

_____

_____

_____

_____

_____

How did you execute your plan?

_____

_____

_____

_____

What is the result of your efforts?

_____

_____

_____

_____

_____

Chapter Four

Feel: No Feel, No Heal

•

"There are people in your life who've come and gone, they've let you down, you know they've hurt your pride. Better put it all behind you, because life goes on. You keep carrying that anger, it'll eat you up inside...but I think it's about forgiveness, forgiveness. Even if, even if, you don't love me anymore."

—Don Henley

FEEL: NO FEEL, NO HEAL

Everything You Do Is Based On Feelings

Don't underestimate the power of your feelings. It's a mistake many people who have suffered emotional trauma make, and it's one that I'm going to help you avoid. Feelings or emotions (I will use the terms interchangeably) are the basis for every action you take. Whether you belly up to the bar at happy hour, spend hours on social media, stay glued to the rec room TV on football Sundays, or make it a point to hit the gym, it's all about how you feel. In fact, you are trying to control your feelings in a positive way. Feelings are why you travel twelve hours across the country on Thanksgiving to see your grandkids' smiling faces; feelings are why Tom Brady chases another Super Bowl ring instead of retiring and resting comfortably on his laurels; feelings are why that troubled kid bullies your kid; and feelings are why your kid considered suicide as an option after being the object of a bully's harassment. Feelings are why Nick Wallenda walks a tightrope across the Niagara and why your uncle attempts marriage again for the fifth time. And feelings are why Vietnam veterans will not talk about their time "in country."

Let me tell you about three Vietnam veterans that I treated. All three had suffered severe and extremely traumatic experiences, resulting in symptoms of PTSD. As a reminder, your experiences may be less intense, but your mission remains the same: remember your story in detail, feel your feelings fully, express and release these feelings, and finally, reframe your story in a positive way that encourages you to thrive. These three gentlemen presented with powerful feelings that overwhelmed them. They were stuck in pain, shame, fear, and hopelessness. When we met, each man was living his life doing everything he could possibly do to avoid confronting and experiencing these feelings.

Trauma Is Maintained by the Avoidance of Feelings (Mr. Avoidance)

Johnny was a truly nice man, the kind of guy who if you needed something, he would be happy to help you if he could. He was a hard worker and a good father to his three daughters; he loved them and his wife with every fiber of his being. But nights were an endless source of hell for Johnny. He checked and rechecked his locked doors many times throughout the night and patrolled the house like a night watchman on the brink of a battle front. Even though his psychiatrist prescribed him enough Xanax to tranquilize a Clydesdale, when Johnny did go down to sleep, he didn't go down for very long. You see, Johnny had a secret—something he had never told anyone—a secret that he carried with him for more than twenty years. Johnny's secret involved the cruel treatment of a young Vietnamese girl who was captured, used for sexual gratification, and then blown to pieces for the entertainment of three deranged men, all of whom were Johnny's superiors. They threatened him and promised dire consequences if he told what he had witnessed, and he never breathed a word of it until he shared the story with me. Instead, he held onto the feelings, including his horror at witnessing something so inhumane and his rage at seeing how people cheapen human life. But perhaps the worst of Johnny's feelings went beyond the horror of the rapes and murder. Johnny felt powerless, emasculated, ineffectual, and to borrow the word that was employed most often in his self-description, "cowardly."

Johnny hated feeling as if he were less than a man. At work, no one knew why he had a propensity for volunteering for all the dangerous missions, seeing as how he had three young children. Somewhere in the back of Johnny's mind was a death wish. He had decided against actively taking his life, as he loved his children and did not want to bring his shame upon them. Nonetheless, should he be killed in a dangerous mission at work, he thought that would be far less devastating to his children and would at last offer him the respite he so desired after losing his manhood in Vietnam. For Johnny to have any hope of being able to heal, he had to finally deal with those very deep-rooted feelings of shame, emasculation, and self-negation.

Dan had also served time in combat in Vietnam. His story was for more typical than Johnny's, in that he had seen his best friend, or "brother" as he thought of him, be shot through his helmet and die in battle. Dan could only follow how he was trained to deal with such incidents, including staying down and firing back, and when appropriate, dragging his buddy's body out of the heat of the battle and eventually back to where the medics could see to his lifeless body. Unfortunately for Dan, there was no time to process and feel his feelings, let alone work toward saying goodbye to his dear friend.

What stayed with Dan for so many years was the following: after he heard the sound of the fatal bullet penetrating his buddies helmet, Dan could feel a gentle splattering on his right shoulder—his buddy's brain—landing on him like the first heavy drops of a summer rain shower. There was no time, no opportunity, nor any protocol for saying goodbye to his buddy, let alone describing what it was like to have his brother-in-arms' brains splatter on his shoulder. When he returned home, Dan didn't speak of this traumatic incident until he began therapy with me.

Michael's feelings were also very powerful. He was the "point man" one day that ended in a gun battle between his troops and the North Vietnamese. Michael shot a sniper in a tree and could see that the man was eating rice when he died. But he lost three of his friends on that day, though not due to his own actions. Michael's losses created feelings not of emasculation, shame, or horror, but of deep sadness. His responses to those losses struck me as being an ironic style of simultaneous avoidance and prolonged exposure. That is, he drank himself to sleep most nights, again, to avoid the depth of his pain. At the same time, he experienced a nightly ritual of watching the same day described above in detail in his dreams. Night after night, year after year, for more than thirty years, his mind featured the very same dream. Why, you ask? Behavior is purposeful, and his nightly dream celebrated the life of his fallen brethren, who would otherwise have been long forgotten, their contributions to the world rendered all but meaningless. Michael gave them a nightly opportunity to rise again and sacrifice their lives one more time for their country. In this way, he never had to grieve their losses or how they symbolized the 58,000 young men and women who died, according to Michael, in "the most meaningless of wars." As long as Michael could maintain the dream, he would never have to face his feelings. And because of his alcoholism, insomnia, and deep depression, Michael was never successful in any of his efforts at maintaining a healthy relationship.

One thing was certain for him; no woman could ever understand his nightly ritual and his unconscious need to keep his "brothers" alive.

Trauma Is Healed by the Expression and Release of Feelings

Feelings, as above, are the driving force for all you do. Likewise, feelings are why you hold onto something such as an article of clothing, a love note, or an old car when it no longer serves any other purpose. Feelings also contain the key to what memories you keep and cherish, as in an old favorite story of a conquest, or a hilarious tale involving your best friend's coming of age. Telling those stories may only serve to strengthen feelings. The stories may become funnier than they already were, for instance. Telling the story repeatedly may also strengthen your need to maintain the story, as for example if it elicits laughter or compassion from others whenever it is told.

But why would you hold onto painful or traumatic feelings if they robbed you of peace, sleep, or even hope? You wouldn't, not voluntarily. And yet you do, not by embellishing the traumatic story, but by avoiding it. Johnny would never speak about his horror, because to do so would bring his cowardliness to life. If the story was never told, maybe it never happened? And if it did, the fewer people who knew about it, the better. He had considered telling others about what he experienced, but how would others view him after they knew what he had allowed to happen to that girl? Surely, many would question his goodness as a person; he could imagine hearing others asking him, "How could you let that happen to that poor innocent girl?" He often asked himself this question. What did it mean about him as a person? Was this transgression forgivable in God's eyes? Johnny found himself questioning his past often but never spoke about these issues to anyone and chose instead to suffer alone. While he was avoiding the feelings, Johnny could never heal.

Dan remembered that his friend had died, but repressed the details. The fact of his friend's death was terribly sad; the way he had died was horrific. By repressing the splattering of his friend's brain on his shoulder, Dan would never need to experience that horror. But unfortunately, without experiencing the horror, Dan would never heal.

Michael played his movie in his mind every night to revisit his pain in the past. So why wasn't he closer to healing if he was allowing himself access to the worst day of his life? Two reasons: Michael separated himself from his feelings of sorrow and loss by drinking himself into a nightly stupor. He couldn't dream if he couldn't sleep, and he couldn't sleep until he was good and soused. For Michael, excessive alcohol consumption was functional. Logically, if he didn't sleep, he couldn't dream. But since his body required him to sleep whether he wanted to or not, being black-out drunk was a functional solution. Intoxication often prevented the dreams, which in turn prevented the feelings. Secondly, to truly experience his sadness would be to admit (and accept) that his friends were gone, and from Michael's perspective, they had died in vain. To fully feel his sadness was the first step to releasing and letting go. It meant that he was finally accepting the loss of his friends and facing reality for what it truly was. Often people want to "forget and move on," but when forgetting a lost loved one isn't an option, letting go of the pain and hurt is the only alternative. Through feeling your feelings, the ability to release and let go can be achieved.

But feeling your feelings, as dreadful as it may appear to be, is also critical to the healing process. In fact, Johnny, Dan, and Michael all needed to feel—completely feel. Johnny needed to feel his helplessness, as well as his outrage toward his superiors and the "callous US government." He needed to feel the horror of watching a life, many lives actually, destroyed. He needed to feel the "weakness" of watching humans express their personal brokenness by destroying innocence and engaging in a disgrace of their roles and responsibilities. And he needed to feel his powerlessness to stop any of it and the ugliness of having been a part of it. He needed to not circumvent these feelings; he had to feel them fully, express them, and release them. It was then and only then that he could reclaim his life, find meaning, and make a difference, as it was only then that he could reclaim his humanity, his dignity, and his faith. It was the only road to resurrecting Johnny from the ashes, the boy/man who was destroyed in Vietnam.

Dan had to be brought back to the scene of his friend's death. He needed to feel the sensation upon his shoulder and understand that it represented the destruction of life and the demise of a friendship. He needed to feel that in war, life is very cheap, and he needed to experience the senselessness of people dying for a cause unknown. Dan needed to feel all of that to force his way back to a place where life—his own, his family's, and that of others—was no longer cheap and meaningless. He would have to find a way to live as if that were his truth.

As for Michael, I enjoyed offering him an opportunity to amend and finally complete his dream, rather than endlessly watching his "dream movie." We created an ending where his three brave friends were celebrated and appreciated—and their lives validated—in a ceremony that Michael devised to honor his fallen veterans. In that way, there was no need to continue the dream. The alcohol, although instrumental as his "sleep aid," then needed to be addressed as a problem unto itself. As of the date of this writer, Michael is still unwilling to commit to a program to address his alcoholism.

For these men and for you, healing requires feeling your trauma to its fullest in order to release the hold it has on you. It is the only way to release the trauma(s), take your life back from the unfinished pain in the past, and return the responsibility for happiness to you.

Questions for Comprehension

—

What are the three best ideas that you gleaned from this chapter?

_____

_____

_____

_____

_____

What type of action do you believe is necessary to help actualize these ideas?

_____

_____

_____

_____

_____

How did you execute your plan?

_____

_____

_____

_____

_____

What is the result of your efforts?

_____

_____

_____

_____

_____

Chapter Five

Express: Let the Water Flow

"Let me take a long last look before we say goodbye."

—Don Henley

EXPRESS: LET THE WATER FLOW

The twelve steps of Alcoholics Anonymous (AA) are the foundation of countless stories of sobriety. These time-tested pearls of wisdom have stood unchanged since Bill Wilson and Dr. Bob Smith co-authored them in 1935.[39] To get sober, you must (1) admit there is a problem that you can't handle, (2) acknowledge that there is a force greater than you that can help, and (3) surrender your problem to that force. Simply put, those are the first three steps of the AA program.

But then something interesting develops in steps four and five—you must write your "fearless moral inventory" (basically how you have mucked up everything in your life and everyone else's around you) and then express these painful confessions to someone you trust, usually your sponsor.

Why read it aloud when it's absolutely nobody's business? Because again, it is the feeling and expression of emotion that allows for release, and ultimately, healing. Stated in the negative, **you will not heal your**

pain in the past without the expression of your story (feelings included)—every nasty little bit of it.

Here is the secret to why psychotherapy often works so well: expressing emotional pain is cathartic and healing, especially if you are willing to release the pain, as you'll see in the next chapter.

It Ain't Real Until You Express It

Danielle sat in silence for just over thirty-two minutes, a record in my office. Never at a loss for words, she told me the story about her uncle, who had molested her at age seven. Eventually she stated, "He put it up to my mouth."

"Put what up to your mouth?" Of course, I knew.

"You know."

"It's important that you tell me everything."

"I can't."

"You can. We are going to put this away today."

Then came the long period of silence while she battled with herself for the courage to verbalize it.

Why did I require such detail? It was not to be sadistic. Unless all the details are shared, they can remain unacknowledged and unconscious and will therefore retain their emotional power. In fact, *without ever stating the details of the event, it is as if those parts of the story never happened.* All the details of the horror must be remembered, felt, expressed, and released to put the horror away for good. Danielle didn't want to say the word "penis" aloud, because the moment she did, it became real.

I've expressed this before, but it bears repeating: for something to become real requires a witness, an interpersonal context. Expressing what happened in front of a mirror or crying yourself to sleep are both ineffective for the same reason. Yes, you need to express your pain, but doing it in front of someone is required. Understandably, Danielle didn't want to say that her uncle forced her to perform fellatio upon him.

When she finally said the word (and finished the story), she began to cry and expressed the horror of her victimization. She even forgave me for not allowing her to skip over the expression of that word.

There's an old expression you may have heard: share your joy with someone and it doubles, share your sorrow and it is cut in half. That's not a scientific fact, but like a lot of adages, it's the wisdom of accumulated experience. The expression of self to another is the cornerstone of human connection, validation, intimacy, and as with the client above, healing.

The expression of your feelings to another person is what (hopefully) separates intimate relationships from acquaintances. It also separates psychotherapy from a casual chat with your cat. The research continues to support that expressing feelings to someone safe and validating is very healing. Or in the words of Karyn Hall, PhD, the Psychology Today Director of the Dialectical Behavioral Therapy Center in Houston, Texas[40], "Validation is the recognition and acceptance of another person's thought's feelings, sensations, and behaviors as understandable."

Rick's Story

Rick was a sixty-three-year-old radiologist with an alcohol problem. The Penn State scandal of 2011 involved the sexual abuse of boys by a football coach, defensive coordinator Jerry Sandusky. This event triggered flashbacks and nightmares for Rick about his middle school experiences, involving, of all things, a traveling magician.

When Rick was twelve, his school hired a magician who traveled cross-country entertaining students by pulling rabbits out of hats and sawing people in half. But there is always a trick that requires the participation of a volunteer, and Rick was chosen. He was the lucky one, or so he thought. He excitedly approached the stage, smiling as if he just won some "never have to do another homework assignment" contest. He was placed in a box and made to disappear, reappear in a different box, then disappear again. Rick was just as entertained by his role in the performance as the audience was.

When the trick ended, the magician held Rick's hand high in the air in obvious acclaim. Rick experienced the proudest moment of his young life. As Rick was about to walk back to his seat, the magician whispered, "If you want to know how it's done, come backstage after the show."

Backstage, the magician stalled for time, making sure that everyone had left the building. When they were alone, the magician went into his truck and removed pictures of naked young boys Rick's age and younger and showed them to Rick. Rick became nauseous and wanted to escape. He was told to pull his trousers down and bend over as the magician spat upon his hands. The pain of anal penetration, he confessed, was the worst physical pain of his life. The act was over very quickly, as rapists are often extremely aroused by the forbidden circumstances. Rick was reduced to a puddle of tears, humiliated, broken, violated, disgusted. Before he could pull up his pants and escape, the magician got in his face one more time and told him, "If you ever tell anybody, I will kill your entire family including your dog. Got it?" Rick nodded. "Now go!"

Rick took a different way home, as if that would somehow change what had happened. One question stuck with him: "How did he know I have a dog?"

Rick spent the evening weeping and scrubbing himself in the shower, "trying to remove the stench of the rape." He kept the story secret for fifty-one years.

I promised Rick that we would finally make peace with this horrible memory. The next week, we used the guided imagery technique where Rick could watch the entire abuse scene from a seat in an imaginary movie theater. He was asked to play the movie in its entirety, from the moment he sat in the middle school auditorium until the endless shower and eventual tearful sleep.

After reviewing and watching every detail, I asked Rick to enter the movie at his current age, introduce himself to young Rick, and grab him by the shoulders, and to encourage him and tell him how proud he was of him, how well he had turned out, how it wasn't his fault, and how he could finally let this go forever. He spent a long time in that movie, sobbing on my couch, imagining himself comforting young Rick. At that point, we went into the alley behind our imaginary movie theater and Rick destroyed the movie.

He would never need to watch it, feel it, or suffer in shame again. The next session was two weeks later, and I asked Rick to summarize the effect: "It was the second worst 45 minutes of my life (repeating the rape story) followed by the best fifteen minutes of my life (the time spent with young Rick)." His mind was at last free.

Two weeks later, Rick brought me in a painting—a copy of Michelangelo's "Rebellious Servant," that the original of which hangs in the Louvre in Paris. The painting depicts a shackled slave—his hands cuffed behind his back—breaking from his bondage. Rick said, "This is what you have done for me, I am finally out of bondage." The original painting in Paris is worth untold millions. But to me, the copy Rick shared is priceless.

Oh, one more thing: one month later, Rick joined AA and quit drinking. He's now been sober for more than five years.

Methods of Expressing and Letting Go

Over more than thirty-two years as a psychologist, I have facilitated countless sessions of facing trauma and healing by relying upon the five components of the Fritz: Remember, Feel, Express, Release (Let go), Reframe. I am convinced these steps are the ticket to healing from all types of pain in the past, from Mother Nature's vengeance to human cruelty; and from the death of loved ones to the emotional scars of automobile accidents. Whatever the outstanding pain, trauma, or loss, the Fritz works.

How you employ these five steps varies according to the individual and her capacity and willingness to express and release her pain. A substantial percentage of trauma survivors need only to share their stories and the concomitant pain and tears to release the horror once and for all. For those people, merely fetching the ugly story from the pile of unfinished hurt and trauma and sharing it slowly, accurately, and painfully will suffice. There is no need to piggyback another closure technique upon this one.

Suzanne was one such person. After a childhood of being molested by two family members, Suzanne quickly learned that men were going to take what they wanted, whether she agreed or not. She learned as a teen that if she couldn't beat them, she had to join them, and began a life of desperate promiscuity and love-seeking, trading her body and self-respect for the empty promise of love and security. And so began a fifty-year journey to find love and self-acceptance, repeatedly turning to chemicals like alcohol, nicotine, benzodiazepines, and sleep aids to slow down her ailing nervous system. Grossly underweight and fragile at age 68, she was referred by her primary care physician for what was described as "moderate to severe depression." Psychotherapy was as simple as giving Suzanne a safe place to express her story. She shared every last account of men behaving badly in the name of sexuality. Suzanne responded with a willingness to give herself again and again in the hope that someone would emerge as her savior, someone to care for, cherish and protect her, rather than use and discard her.

I wondered if there was a bottom to her painful well of stories of abuse. After endless tales of sadness and hurt, I wanted to yell, "Why? Why did you keep allowing this? You were no longer a victim, you were a volunteer! Why?" But I kept my mouth shut and let her continue weekly therapy as she related one terrible story after another, hoping that there would one day be an end, that expressing and releasing would prove as therapeutic for Suzanne as it had for other clients.

Then three events took place: first, Suzanne finally finished her painful stories—she had, at least, exhausted the supply. This completion as well as depletion of her memory bank of the horror stories made a significant impact on her depressive symptoms and allowed her to gradually redefine her worth and status as a woman.

Secondly, Suzanne met Brian, a man who was struggling with his own issues, including late stage cancer and chronic obstructive pulmonary disease (COPD). Brian thought Suzanne was an angel from heaven and told her so in poems, cards, and flowers. She felt as if Brian was the first man who had ever truly loved her. All he wanted was to be with her, and she believed him. They shared two months of "true love" together before Brian finally succumbed to cancer.

As difficult as Brian's death was for Suzanne—she had finally found love but then had lost it almost as quickly—it satisfied a deep need for a man who adored her for the woman she was.

She smiled and cried at the mere mention of Brian. Even with his broken and decaying body, he was somehow able to convey to Suzanne that she was worth all the love in the world. Now that she had finally expressed and released her toxic stories of hurt and shame, she was prepared to receive kindness from a caring human being, a man who loved her. For Suzanne, at least, there was renewed peace and self-respect.

Two months after Brain's death, a third significant event took place: Suzanne died, a grateful woman with her mission accomplished. I can only hope there is an opportunity to reunite with Brian.

THE GOODBYE LETTER

The expression and release of painful feelings is curative. Once painful feelings are expressed and released, no need exists to hold on to them. One of my personal favorite techniques to help my clients release the pain and anguish associated with trauma is the goodbye letter. The goodbye letter works well in a wide variety of situations because it can be used in association with any type of pain in the past. As discussed in chapter one, Fritz Perls emphasized the importance of finishing "unfinished" business as critical for healing, and this belief led to his development of Gestalt psychology.[33] Writing a "goodbye letter" addresses the feeling of "if only I could have told him/her this..." or of "I'm ready to let this pain go and be released so I can move forward." Saying goodbye formally, in writing, helps people release and let go of whatever it is that needs to be released.

Other famous psychotherapists who have also endorsed the technique of letter writing for closure include Syd Simon, Susan Forward, and Robert Ackerman. Ackerman, an author and lecturer best known for his work with Adult Children of Alcoholics (ACOA)[41], suggested that a four-part letter works best for toxic emotions present since childhood: (1) What happened? (2) How did it feel to be me at the time? (3) How has it affected me since then? (4) What am I doing now to let go? For the sake of clarity, from here on out I'll discuss the four steps of the goodbye letter and then work through an example for grief-stricken individuals, as well as an example for those who were traumatized themselves.

If you're grief-stricken, writing a goodbye letter is a powerful method to express and release pain while also providing you, the letter writer, with a unique opportunity to close the chapter on your beloved's life and to tell your beloved whatever you wanted to get off your chest.

The first step, simply enough, is to detail the events in full. If you are the spouse, for instance, this can be several pages of how the two of you met, that cheesy pickup line, your first date, how she or he rocked your world, spoiled your dog, backed over your flower bed, charmed the socks off you grandmother, helped you raise the children, and cared for you while I was going through cancer treatment, etc. For the death of a child, this can be the never-ending ebb and flow of worry and excitement about their birth, the relief when they were healthy, their first words, steps, and Christmas, their first piano recital, graduating high school, college, etc. Regardless of who passes, this step ends in the shock and horror that occurred when the beloved person actually passed.

Step two falls in line naturally; it begins with how the death of the loved one felt. It's a beautiful opportunity to recite how their existence profoundly, completely, and permanently altered your life. The tears that fall in the first and second step are the bittersweet tears of joy and sorrow. The joy, of course, is the reliving of many of the happiest times in your life together. The sorrow, needless to say, is that those times are no more—you'll never hear her staccato laugh, pick up the fallen evidence of his midnight cookie siege, have your emotional rock to support you, or form new memories together. Writing what you remember and hold so dear may morph into a beautiful memoir, besides being therapeutic.

The third step goes into detail about how the beloved's premature departure from this planet has affected you since then. Much like a boat's passing, even long after the death of a loved one, the ripples can still be felt and need to be expressed as well: the long nights filled with tears, the difficulties finding joy, the negative feelings (profound sadness, guilt), the longing for just one phone call to heaven.

The fourth and final step of the goodbye letter is communicating what you're doing now to say goodbye to (and let go of) the pain. Of the four steps, this is the one most often skipped by letter writers. Why? Because saying goodbye is so final. It is never easy to admit and accept that your loved one will not be returning. You can more easily write fifteen pages extolling the joyous half-century relationship yet avoid the expression of the last half page that allows your loved one permission to leave this world behind. Of course, that makes sense, but without the goodbye, there is no acceptance and ultimately no healing. Many a widow makes that same discovery when she finally bravely donates her late husband's clothing to Goodwill. When the garments are released, she feels an unburdening, a detachment, and the cathartic release of acceptance. It represents the release of the loved one as a physical entity, as well as making peace with the notion that this person will not be back.

Writing the Goodbye Letter After Trauma

The goodbye letter for those of you who have been traumatized is a much different exercise than the one for grief over the loss of a loved one. The first step of "what happened" is not a celebration of a shared life of loving partnership. Instead, you must recall what the perpetrator of the trauma did, in agonizing detail. This part of the letter documents the part of your life that has been buried for years to protect you from the horrors of abuse, incest, rape, and betrayal, as well as "lesser" events such as being shamed or treated indifferently by a parent or being bullied by an older sibling— whatever comprises the content of your pain in the past. The goal for the first step of what happened is simple to understand but difficult to express:

the greater the detail, the greater the immersion into the pain, and therefore the greater the opportunity for release and healing.

Second, express how it felt to be you at the time. Again, the greater the depth of feelings that you discuss, the greater the potential for healing. In the Feeling chapter, I emphasized the need to feel your feelings fully. It's especially important as part of this exercise. All the feelings that have been trapped in your memory must be felt and expressed for release to occur. Horror, fear, hopelessness, vulnerability, panic, impending doom, and thoughts of death or suicide are all common emotions felt by the traumatized and all need to be written and included in this letter. Tears are often an integral part of expressing the pain and horror.

Step three—how this has affected you since then—expresses how your youthful innocence may have been stolen, how your ideas about love and family were permanently stained, or how the world became a dangerous place. In this part of the letter, share how this trauma(s) "robbed me of my naïve smile and replaced it with a look of fear and mistrust and with avoidance of eye contact. Mine is a countenance of shame, my eyes expressionless, dead, no longer conveying a promise of things to come." These second and third steps of the letter allow you the opportunity to express in writing the deepest of human agony and attach words to feelings and sensations that have been virtually indescribable to this point. By expressing and releasing the pain, you can and will achieve healing.

For the trauma survivor, there is nothing more attractive than saying goodbye to the worst thing you've ever been through. Consider what it would be like to rise in the morning without the trauma providing the rude awakening; or the pleasure of living an entire day without a close-up of the perpetrator's evil countenance; or the possibility of shutting your eyes at bedtime knowing you will not experience nocturnal flashbacks and heart-thumping nightmares.

Tamika was a twenty-two-year-old when she made her first therapy appointment. Her story was right out of a movie: Middle-aged man abducts nineteen-year-old girl at gunpoint and holds her hostage for three days in his dark apartment. Tamika was repeatedly raped, threatened, and mocked until she found an opportunity to escape. Two years later, she realized that instead of getting better, she was more under the control of her seventy-two-hour "private hell" than she had been one month after the abduction. "After all this time, why am I not improving?"

By now, you can predict my response to Tamika. "Time doesn't heal; you must remember, feel, express, and release your story. I'm going to need you to share every last detail of your experience until we can finally finish the nightmare..."

Tamika spoke in generalities, and I responded, "Please share all of the details with me." It sounds sadistic, I know, but to repeat myself, if she talked around the abduction, skimmed over the rapes, and recited the facts of her Hollywood escape without tearfully expressing the emotions...you guessed it, she'd never ever heal.

This was a challenge for Tamika because it required her to articulate extremely delicate and fragile emotions. Tamika cried and at one point sobbed uncontrollably when she was asked whether she had thought she'd ever make it out alive. Her recitation of these difficult details lasted for approximately three minutes, but these minutes seemed like forever to Tamika. She was expressing and releasing the greatest terror she had experienced in her entire life. But having expressed the fear so intensely, she didn't have to revisit it in her dreams or hold onto it during the empty spaces in her days.

My questions were open-ended and encouraged her to share everything pertinent to her experience. "Is there more?" "What was the worst part of that aspect (story)?" "How did you feel when you heard him say that?" "Where did you draw your strength from during that moment?"

And when she cried, I reminded her, "Let it all out. It's finally over. It's okay. Pour it all out. You made it, you survived. Now you will get your life back."

I asked Tamika to write a goodbye letter to her perpetrator in order to eliminate his power over her, his presence in her life, and his dark shadow over her future. The goal, as always, was closure—to put this terrible experience away for good and replace the dread, the fear, and the shame with confidence, a sense of pride, and a resolve to make a difference. Tamika responded with the following letter:

> *"I forgive you. Not for what you did, but for who and what you are. No longer will I carry with me all of those memories and ravaged emotions; they serve me no purpose and only show that you are still in control. No longer will I awake to the sight of your face and cry in fear, cringing at the mere thought of what happened. All of the energy I've given to you over the past twenty-two months—I now take it back for myself. You have been the focus of my life for almost two years, and that is too much time. You have taken the one thing from me that I held sacred and treasured most. I will not give you any more than that. My hopes of revenge have long since faded, along with the anger. I refuse to feel defeated, for I have not given up. I simply refuse to expend any unnecessary energy on something that will only cause me pain. I don't have time for it. My life must continue. I must pick up where I was before you came into the picture—as the happy, ambitious, hardworking, girl I once was. My goals are once again in view, no longer clouded over with visions of pain. You have taken a great deal from me, but if I force myself to look closely, I can also see what I have gained; most importantly, the ability to overcome. There*

is no longer a question in my mind of, "Will he control me forever?" The answer is no—I have won.

So goodbye. You will receive no more from me. You are no longer with me. The rest of my journey will be traveled alone, with the company and presence only of those I love. This is the last of it—my final farewell."

GUIDED IMAGERY

This is the very best and most effective technique for emotional trauma, but it's likely that your therapist doesn't use it and may not even have heard of it. Why? It's neglected in most mainstream psychology programs, as is Fritz Perls' Gestalt Theory. It's time to rediscover this wonderful technique.

What is guided imagery? Like hypnosis, it is merely relaxed concentration and focus on an imaginary story. It's also a way to gain closure on the trauma you suffered by watching it (as if it were a film in a theater) one more time and finishing it.

Guided imagery can be used for many purposes, including:

- Saying goodbye to people who have died and making peace with their passing.

- Releasing losses that have lingered for decades and accepting them.

- Bidding farewell to (and confronting) a deceased perpetrator of a trauma.

Much like hypnosis, guided imagery can be used to see parts of an unfinished memory up close and then release those most treacherous memories. With guided imagery, a fresh opportunity exists to say goodbye, hear 'I'm sorry' or apologize, and have someone else accept your apology, and reconnect, etc.

Not surprisingly, this type of imagery is often used by sports psychologists to help their athletes improve, from ice skating routines to a golfer's putting. To see something with your mind's eye and your body relaxed helps convince you that the movie in your head is or can be real. Moreover, it feels entirely real, allowing your nervous system to respond as if it were.

One of the more fascinating research studies involving guided imagery had nothing at all to do with healing or trauma, but rather focused on 6th grade students shooting basketball free throws. Children were assessed on their free throw shooting and then assigned into one of three groups. One group did nothing for six weeks; the second group shot basketball free throws daily for six weeks; and the third group **imagined** shooting basketball free throws using guided imagery daily for six weeks. The three groups were then retested. Predictably, the first group did not improve during their six-week stint of no basketball. Group number 2 improved their percentage of baskets by 23 percent due to their daily practice—no big surprise. But the guided imagery group, who hadn't touched a basketball for six weeks except in their minds, improved by 22 percent! Can you really improve a skill merely by practicing that skill only in the privacy of your head?[42] Indeed.

And that's the beauty of guided imagery. Seeing something in your imagination only tricks the nervous system into believing that the event was real, or at least felt that way. As a clinician who has experienced the power of this technique to help deal with pain in the past, I want you to become familiar with what it is and how to use it.

How to Conduct a Guided Imagery

Here's a startling but valid statement about guided imagery: it often produces more healing and closure in one session than what a traumatized individual has managed on her own over decades.

How do I conduct guided imagery? The term "guided" implies that someone (hopefully an experienced therapist, not your hairdresser) is available to facilitate the experience. Your job is to follow along with the suggestions, creating in your mind a video as immersive as real experience. Here is what you would experience if you came to me for guided imagery treatment.

To begin, I try to get you to relax. The goal is to have your entire body relaxed from head to toe. First, you use progressive muscle relaxation to dissolve tension anywhere in your body. Tighten each muscle group, hold it for five seconds, then release. Once flexed, each muscle group returns to a lower state of resting tension. After that, move on to deep breathing. You inhale to a count of three, hold your breath for a few seconds, then exhale to a count of five. Changing the ratio of oxygen to carbon dioxide in the blood stimulates an additional relaxation response.

Next, get in a comfortable position and close your eyes. You may be seated or reclined. Bring your attention to your breathing, but this time, breathe naturally. If I observe behavioral evidence of tension, such as fidgeting, frowning, or signs of discomfort, I may ask you to climb down a flight of stairs with each step representing a deeper state of relaxation. Sometimes I ask you to imagine being injected with a powerful tranquilizer and to visualize the tranquilizer as a blue substance that can be seen moving through your body. As it travels, the blue color replaces a hot neon pink color that represents stress, tension, pain, trauma, or anything else requiring release. Once the blue color permeates your entire body, I ask you if any part of your body is still tense. If so, the tranquilizer then travels to that area.

Once you're completely relaxed, I ask you to imagine a door. Inside is a movie theater where you may watch some tragic scene unfold on the big screen. You open the door and are seated. I suggest that a remote control appears, allowing you to play, pause, fast-forward, rewind, and stop the experience. You are in complete control of the movie.

Next, I ask you to watch the entire movie from beginning to end. When the movie is over, I invite you at your current age to enter the movie and provide comfort and solace to the younger version of yourself who is suffering in that same scenario. The older version may ask a rapist or molester to leave, for example, or provide comfort to the younger version of yourself. After an ugly scene or trauma, I may have the projectionist offer a DVD of the movie for you to take out back and destroy, symbolizing that the event is over.

In cases of grief, guided imagery requires opening the door that leads into a living room, into a favorite cabin in the woods, or into the kitchen where the person grew up, and so on. Here, a conversation is created between you and the person for whom you are grieving, perhaps someone lost in an accident, an estranged child who died without reconciliation, a spouse who died suddenly, or anyone with whom you have unfinished business. I speak for the deceased individual in order to provide some sense of closure. This always involves putting things that are still hurtful in a better place. Examples include apologies for abuse or betrayal and expressions of love to you from someone who could not communicate it well. It may also include you expressing your own hurt, anger, or rage toward someone who in some way mistreated or abandoned you, as well as acknowledgment from the perpetrator of the trauma. Finally, you may also use this technique to express appreciation and gratitude to a loved one that was not fully expressed while the person was alive.

Why Does Guided Imagery Work?

All human relationships are naturally unfinished works-in-progress. Parents are expected to nurture. Children are expected to grow up. When a relationship is complete, expectations are satisfied. A good son transitions from being a good man to being a good father. Traumatic events, though, interrupt the natural flow of your life events and produce experiences of loss. These events are then consciously or unconsciously avoided and often sealed off from your conscious experience. As such, their treatment involves: (1) making the traumatic event accessible to conscious awareness through guided imagery, and (2) modifying the context or adding something that completes the relationship or finishes the trauma, thus helping you move to a better place. Once again, what is experienced in imagery is processed as reality by the nervous system and feels real to you.

Other Assorted Techniques

While guided imagery and letter writing are by far my two favorite closure exercises, other ways exist to let go of and finish something painful from the past.

For instance, one young man, after realizing that his father was gone and most likely not returning, decided he needed to grieve his loss. I offered him the opportunity to participate in either letter writing or guided imagery. The client wanted neither. Instead, he suggested he could sit in the woods banging on his bongos until he was able to release his biological father. Bongo therapy? I didn't see why not. The client took care of saying goodbye to his father as if it were some primitive ritual near a campfire in the clearing of the forest. Who would argue with the results? It was a one-time deal for my client, and I was schooled in the importance of allowing clients to take the lead in their treatment even when they choose a technique that may be outside of my experience.

My point isn't that everyone should try Bongo therapy, but that people often have methods that are uniquely viable for themselves. Jeremy grew up in a rough, inner-city neighborhood in Newark, New Jersey. He didn't have a father to look up to, but he did have an older cousin, Leroy, who was his unofficial mentor. Leroy had no relationship with drugs, alcohol, or cigarettes. As a result, Jeremy was also clean when it came to dangerous chemicals—not bad for an adolescent on the wrong side of the city tracks.

But one day some gangbangers drove up to the boys on a city side street, and someone yelled, "Just f***ing do it!" Seconds later, the gun-toting guy blew Leroy away with a series of shots. Jeremy sat on the curb yelling, "No, Leroy, nooooo! Don't die, Leroy! Please don't die! Somebody help!"

Within minutes, Leroy was dead, the victim of a drive-by shooting. And sixteen-year-old Jeremy was forced to face his future without the person he most looked up to. Ironically, this was the worst thing that had ever happened to him, and he was forced to deal with it without his mentor. His mother, horrified by her nephew's death and concerned about Jeremy's future, decided to move to Florida to get away from the inner city and gain a fresh start on things. She thought therapy might help him.

Rapping Up the Loss

By the time I met Jeremy, he had already written two notebooks full of rap songs about his life, many of them about or dedicated to cousin Leroy. Though I'm not knowledgeable about rap music (as I prefer M&M's to Eminem), Jeremy's lyrics were powerful, moving, and well-written. Jeremy didn't want to say goodbye to Leroy but was tired of hurting so much from reliving the tragedy.

So in keeping with his love for his mentor, his passion for rapping, and the power of the Fritz, I asked him to write (at least) one more rap song that would memorialize Leroy's life, keeping his positive legacy intact, but allowing him to pass on to the next world. I asked Jeremy to retain the positive gifts from his cousin and use them to make a difference as a way to honor Leroy. I also asked that he live his life in victory, not resentment and defeat, because although Leroy's life was too short, his contributions would remain as long as Jeremy did. The result of my request was a beautiful poem, one that brought tears to my otherwise stoic eyes, that praised Leroy for his love and then blessed him on his continued journey to the hereafter. As he read that rap to me, I could tell there was something very different—Jeremy had hope for the first time since I had met him. How? He had figured out a way to honor his fallen cousin, hold on to his goodness, and yet let go of the need to dwell in chronic rage and hopelessness. And his method of gaining closure? Inner-city rap.

Other Techniques to Express and Release

All faiths espouse teachings on the afterlife, whether the promise is reincarnation, resting in peace, or "many mansions," accompanied by rituals that are designed to aid in grieving and accepting the loss of the departed.

In the Jewish faith, for instance, people are celebrated at their death with "a beautiful, structured approach to mourning that involves three stages... The loss is forever, but the psychological, emotional, and spiritual healing that takes place at every stage is necessary and healthy."[43]

The goal is to afford the opportunity for the survivors to deeply honor the departed, sufficiently grieve the loss (say goodbye), and return to life with the capacity to experience peace and joy once again, finally gaining some closure on the life and death of the departed.

And isn't closure one of the purposes of funerals? Celebrations of life? Memorial services? The Vietnam Memorial? The Holocaust Museum? The Civil War Memorial? Cemeteries?

Healing from trauma or loss requires feeling the pain of the experiences and then expressing the pain in some form or another in an effort to release the person or trauma to a place where it is now acceptable to continue peacefully, hopefully, and positively with life. This is the purpose of employing the Fritz.

The importance of expression cannot be overstated; it allows your healing to begin. Expression is the removing of the splinter, which allows the process to progress. Without it, of course, you are stuck in your pain in the past. However, once your pain is fully remembered, felt, and expressed, the process of releasing and reframing can begin.

Questions for Comprehension

—

What are the three best ideas that you gleaned from this chapter?

_____

_____

_____

_____

_____

What type of action do you believe is necessary to help actualize these ideas?

_____

_____

_____

_____

_____

How did you execute your plan?

_____

_____

_____

_____

What is the result of your efforts?

_____

_____

_____

_____

Chapter Six

Release: Release for Peace

•

*Life is a series of hellos and goodbyes, I'm afraid
it's time for goodbye again.*
—Billy Joel

LET IT GO: RELEASE FOR PEACE

As long as you're still breathing, there remains hope for healing. This doesn't mean time heals all wounds. All time does is pass; healing requires the volitional act of letting go. Of course, people often do gradually let go over time—as in most divorces, for instance—and so time erroneously receives credit.

You've read about people who needed to let go of molestation, rape, betrayals, and combat atrocities. These people sought to remove one or more horrible incident(s) from their minds but could not because the horror had not been digested successfully (remembered, felt, expressed, released).

Letting go is tough. Awareness of this difficulty is useful, providing insight into how deep the hold of a given trauma can be. As I've emphasized, people refuse to let go because to do so constitutes an acceptance of the death of a loved one or the acceptance of a situation that is deemed to be unacceptable.

Randi's Story

Unlike a lot of trauma survivors, Randi could easily tell her story from start to finish; she relished the telling. Randi had been married to Dr. Dave for twenty-one years, had helped put him through medical school, had raised his four boys, and had endured an affair he'd had with a pretty young "Miss Bimbo," then forgave him and welcomed him back, no questions asked. Shortly thereafter, Randi watched Dave walk out of her life for good. Eventually, he divorced Randi and ultimately married "Miss Bimbo."

It's a familiar story especially among affluent men like doctors: the first wife is dumped along the way and replaced with a younger second wife. Once the doctor is successful at his craft and capable of wooing the younger lady with his prestige, his money, and his paternal concern and guidance, he takes action. The first wife is left holding the bag (the kids, the first house, and its memories). She's also mired in the painful questions, "Did he ever love me? Was it all a lie? What could I have done differently? Was it my fault? How could he do this to his children? Doesn't he know divorce ruins lives? Is he so narcissistic that he can't think about anyone else but himself and Miss Bimbo's fake boobies?"

The hurt, the betrayal, the destruction of plans, the rejection and replacement, the fear of starting over—Randi had an endless supply of feelings to express. She could remember the details of the betrayal and abandonment, as well as the myriad broken promises. She could feel and express her feelings and did so time and again, to no avail. There was no healing for Randi.

Why not? Because the mere *expression* of emotional pain is not always curative; in fact, for Randi, it required not only expression of her pain, but ultimately its release. But to release pain is ultimately to let go, and letting go equals forgiving. Simply put, in order to recover herself and the compassionate, caring person she had once been, Randi would have to choose to let go of what Dr. Dave and Miss Bimbo had done. She couldn't hold onto the pain if she ever hoped to feel good again. This is what I told her.

"Well, that makes no sense," she said, flabbergasted that as a psychologist, I failed to "understand that I can never let go of my hatred for them because that would condone the betrayal. Betrayal is never okay, Dr. Cortman, can't you see that? If I forgave them—and I never, ever will—then I'd be saying that betrayal is okay with me. Of course, I can't do that! I won't do that."

But Randi's stance, as convincing as it sounded, was deeply flawed.

Forgiveness, which is best defined as letting go, never condones the bad behavior of the offending party. Forgiveness is not revenge, nor aiming to get even. Nor is it forgetting. It is merely releasing the pain, so it loses its power to dominate your life with its seething animosity. Most accurately, forgiveness allows you the freedom to live again and to exist without the sting of the trauma dominating your every waking moment. The offending party may also benefit from your forgiveness, but ultimately forgiving someone else, first and foremost, is a gift for yourself.

Randi needed to release her contempt if she were to ever reclaim her life and recapture her purpose. What Dave did may always be wrong in her eyes, but hating him would never correct that wrong. All Randi would accomplish by draping herself in hatred would be to guarantee that *she* would never find happiness again. Ironically, Dave and Miss Bimbo might never feel any adverse effects from her negativity. In fact, by remaining mired in negativity, Randi was only hurting her children and herself. **Hence, the destruction that always seems to follow chronic hatred is self-destruction.**

But Randi's hatred was covering more than just hurt, rejection, and abandonment. By hating him, she wouldn't have to address her fear. If she were to let go of her resentment for her two adversaries, she would have to address her fear of starting her life over again. There would be much less money, so there was a need to get a job for the first time in two plus decades. She would be saddled with the responsibility of raising the four boys as a single mother.

When Randi finally faced these truths, she told me, "I am fifty-seven pounds heavier than when I met Dave. I have four kids and no money—who will ever want me?" Tearfully, she continued, "Will I spend the rest of my life alone?" The accompanying tears this time were expressions of deep sadness and the fear of never being loved again.

At this point, therapy took a decided turn. It was no longer helpful for Randi to waste her energy supply on hating her husband and his lover—it was counterproductive. While she was stewing in her rage, Randi was a miserable, self-pitying ogre that even her boys were beginning to avoid. To recapture any semblance of a life, Randi would need to accept that Dave had moved on and more than likely, was never coming back. She would need to tell herself things that were hurtful and truly hard to accept—he had withdrawn his affection from her account, like a financial transaction, and redeposited those same affections in another woman's account.

She also confessed that in fact, she hadn't been there for him and was no longer impressed by his doctor/hero stories anymore; also, the sex was bad.

Still, Randi needed to process some difficult truths: "Don't I deserve any credit for my years of looking after him and his kids? Is there nothing to be said for our marital vows, you know, sickness and health, richer and poorer, forsaking all others...doesn't that count for anything? I know plenty of other men who never strayed when the marriage wasn't wonderful anymore. They didn't sleep with the first available young thing who showed interest. I guess I just don't get it."

Essentially, both she and Dave had admittedly grown tired of one another and stopped investing energy into the marriage. They were living a very lonely existence, but they had stayed together due to the children until Dave was caught cheating on Randi. As embarrassing as his affair may have been for Dave when Randi found out, in another way, it was a truthful beacon of light cast onto the sham marriage that existed behind closed doors. They had the option of repairing their broken marriage, but Dave wanted none of it. He was ready to move on to something that was fresh, new, and validating for him. This pretty young lady really seemed to like him and found him fascinating, knowledgeable, and even sexy. His goal was not to punish Randi, but it had been years since he had enjoyed her company.

Randi admitted she wouldn't miss the marriage they'd had for the last eight to ten years, it was just unfair that she had been the one to help to launch Dave's career and now some other woman would be reaping the benefits of his success. Sure, there'd be a settlement, and probably some alimony, but her attorney warned her against thinking that she could rely on that to make ends meet. If there were to be exotic vacations, the cruise to Italy they'd talked about for years—all that would be enjoyed by Dave and his new woman, not Randi.

But the toughest task for Randi was mustering the courage to reinvent herself as a single mother, with a new job, new friends, and new activities. It was about rediscovering who she was apart from Dave and blossoming as the intelligent woman she had stopped believing in a long time ago.

Eventually, I asked Randi to write a goodbye letter to Dave—one she'd never mail—detailing her inner experience from the day they'd met until now. I asked her to include the ups and downs of child-rearing, from their most joyous moments together to the darkest hours of loneliness and despair. I also asked her to own whatever was hers, including dropping out of the marriage as she had and her lack of interest in him as a person and a professional. "Be as angry as you need to be," I advised her, "say whatever you need to say, but then we're going to let it all go and send him on his way with Amy—the real person, not a caricature bimbo—and wish them well." Randi needed to thank him for whatever had been good in their shared time—the boys, for instance—and release all other aspects of their lives together. There would be no more hatred, no bitter name-calling, no blasting Dave in front of the kids. It was time to gracefully and mindfully pick up the pieces and recreate her life, step by step.

Randi needed about six months of therapy before she realized that in reality, Dave had done her a favor. She was excited to learn that by facing all her fears head-on, she could deal with the aspects of her new life. She loved working out and watching her clothes fall off her body as she lost weight. Most importantly, she liked being able to smile at people genuinely because she had rediscovered that she was a resilient, confident woman who made the world a better place, if only by being her wonderful self.

Randi bravely persevered and forged what any psychologist would consider a happy ending or positive outcome. But notice that I avoided getting into a power struggle with her about the need to forgive (let go). That was deliberate. One of the biggest mistakes a psychologist (or a preacher) can make is to hit the suffering and angry person over the head with the need to forgive. It's the right message, but when sent at the wrong time, it is offensive, insulting, and very invalidating. In fact, it's possibly the best way to lose that client for good—and potentially alienate the sufferer from further help and all well-meaning professionals. Students and grieving family members and friends of the mass shooting in Parkland, Florida, on February 14, 2018, heard that very same message to forgive delivered by a well-meaning minister less than a week after the shooting. Once again, many were offended and insulted when told that their outrage needed to morph into instant forgiveness. This was an overwhelming suggestion to those intimately affected by the shooting. Again, ultimately forgiveness is the answer, but introducing that less than a week after the shootings is like asking a kindergarten student to forego the ice cream and place the money instead into a trust fund for college. Again, a good message, but inappropriate timing.

If you'll take a moment, let's be clear that the "let go" step is the fourth for a reason—you must fully process your pain in the past by first remembering every detail, feeling all the relevant emotions, and expressing them before you are challenged to let go and say goodbye. In the case of the mass shooter, it is ultimately more about accepting the loss of the beloved than about forgiving the shooter. Just as in Randi's situation, she needed to let go of her marriage to Dave and accept life without him as her husband.

WHEN YOUR PAIN IS SAYING GOODBYE TO A LOVED ONE

Seventy-one-year-old Joe sat in the hot tub with his wife Susan of "three hundred years." They had it all, he figured, good health, plenty of money, three independent, high-functioning adult children, and a brood of grandkids. He'll never forget raising his wine glass to Sue in a grateful toast to a life that appeared successful from anybody's vantage point.

Two weeks later, Joseph Jr. fell off a mountain. Big Joe was brought to his knees in desperation. He lived and relived his hot tub toast to Susan as a defining moment in his life, as if he had placed a fairy-tale curse upon his family by toasting his and their good fortune, and by so doing had infuriated the powers that ruled his universe.

"Joey" junior was dead at age thirty-eight, and now suddenly none of the other successes mattered, not even one bit. More than a year after Joey died, Big Joe sought my help. A highly educated man, he was also very practical in his thinking and curt in his verbal expression. "With no disrespect to you, Dr. Cortman, I doubt you or anyone can help me. The way I see it, unless you can bring back Joey, we are probably wasting our time and Medicare's money." Not one given to wasting our government's resources, I accepted Joe's challenge to join forces with him to see if our combined efforts could make a difference.

Once again, it was less about forgiving someone and more about saying goodbye to Joey. If there's one thing that all human parents seem to agree upon, it's that they should be buried by their children, and never, ever, vice versa. Losing a child at any age, according to Joe, is "unnatural, unfair, tragic, and has a way of making all other aspects of life appear trivial by comparison."

Maybe because Joe and I had such a powerful connection and maybe because he was out of options, he chose to trust me. Trusting me meant that we would need to say goodbye to Joey and to commemorate him by finding meaning for his life and premature death that made sense to his father. No platitudes would do the trick: the idea that "God needed Joey more than you did" was not going to provide peace for Joe.

Guided Imagery

After two months of treatment, I told Joe that I often used a technique—guided imagery—where he would have an opportunity to visit with his son one more time and tell Joey whatever he needed to say. Of course, it would also allow for Joe to hear from Joey, as well.

Tricking your nervous system is the key to guided imagery. Once again, if the mind's eye sees something, real or imagined, it is processed as real by the nervous system. This is why dreams are so powerful. A dream is merely a movie that you write, direct, and star in. Awaken from a dream and you may exclaim, "Oh, my God, that was so real!" You feel frightened, embarrassed, amused, aroused, defeated, or whatever, depending upon the content of the dream. People may ask others if something really happened or whether they only dreamed it.

The goal for Joe was simple: Have Big Joe meet Joey, tell him the words a male parent doesn't easily bestow upon a male child: "I love and miss you. I think about you every day. I am devastated by your loss." etc. Give Joey that same opportunity, and then add the all-important challenges from son to father to recognize the following:

> *"I am well where I am, but I'm not permitted to share any details about the future except that I am happy, and you will be here one day soon. So, we will reconnect one day. Dad, my life on Earth is over, but yours isn't. There is more for you to do and more lives that you must touch. My kids—your grandkids—need you now more than ever. You are never to use me as a reason to give up on life or to be depressed. I will always be close by you, Dad, until that day when we can reunite. You're still in God's hands, and He has purposes for you until the day you join me here. Please know that my death was an accident, but God remakes all human accidents as purposeful according to his will. Oh, and one more thing, I loved you and mom with all my being, and my wife and kids as well, as much as a man can love. My physical separation from you all doesn't change that one bit. Do you think you could tell them how much I loved them, every once in a while, for me?"*

I could tell you how that experience was for Joe and how transformational that one session was for him, but perhaps it's better to have him tell you himself.

> *"I started working with Dr. Cortman in an effort to help me deal with the grief associated with the tragic loss of the life of my thirty-eight-year-old son, who fell to his death in a mountain climbing accident. During our visits, I exhibited the classic symptoms of grief, especially denial, anger, and lack of acceptance. After many visits, Dr. Cortman*

suggested a technique, Guided Imagery, that might help me. During the Guided Imagery process, I felt like I was able to communicate with my son; I felt that he was present with me, and I was able to have a connection with him. The Guided Imagery process acted as a "switch" and helped me to let him go, to say "goodbye" to him. In essence, the use of Guided Imagery brought me peace and helped me to accept my loss."

All of Joe's problems did not magically disappear, of course, with his encounter with Joey. There was still a lot of work to do related to finding meaning in his son's life and death, coping with anxiety related to his own approaching demise, and even forgiving himself for his own imperfections. But there was a peace regarding Joey's death that provided hope that Big Joe's life was worth doing—even without his precious son.

Marc's Story

Like Joey, Marc's thirty-year-old son died accidentally. He had lost his seven-year battle with opiates, and his parents Marc and Nancy were referred to me for grief therapy. I saw them together—once—but never again, until Marc showed up alone, two years later.

"It's the guilt," he told me, "I can't seem to get over... Every day I feel so guilty that my son is dead."

"What did you attempt to do?" I asked.

"That's just it. I tried everything. I talked to him several times every week. I put him in rehab twice and paid for everything. I tried tough love. Geez, I don't know what else a father could have done to save his child. But after everything I did, Matthew is dead."

"So why the guilt, if you did everything a father could do, Marc?"

"Because he still f***ing died! No matter what I tried, he's still dead. I failed to save my own son!"

The tears were buried beneath rage, self-contempt, and as advertised, guilt. But I wasn't having it.

"With all due respect, guilt is not your problem." I knew he would respect me for presenting him with the truth.

"It's not?"

"No, not really. Don't get me wrong. I'm sure you feel horribly bad about Matthew's death. It's easy to see how much you loved him. But guilt is just a cover for the big issue."

"Which is?"

"Grief. You lost your son, Marc, and the sadness is almost immeasurable. The guilt is just a protest—a cover, if you will—for the deep sadness. Let me explain: as long as you continue to feel guilty, you are saying that Matthew's death, somehow, is your fault. You don't have to say goodbye to Matthew. It's as if you are saying that his death is still under protest. It shouldn't have happened. And therefore, you can't release him, because it was all one big mistake."

"Okay, so what do we have to do so I can stop feeling so guilty?"

"You have to say goodbye to Matthew. It's the toughest thing I can ask you to do, but it is the reason you are wallowing in terrible guilt."

Again, I resorted to guided imagery, and again, I trusted myself to speak on behalf of Matthew. I related to Marc that, "You didn't fail me, Dad. In fact, you were the only one that I knew would still talk to me, even when I went back to using after being in rehab. You always tried to help me because you never stopped caring. I could see that, even after I screwed up. No matter what I did, you never stopped loving me, Dad. I can't tell you how much I appreciate that. But Dad, there is a simple answer to the question of what went wrong. I didn't want to stop using the drugs. I liked how they helped me feel better. It's really that simple. You didn't fail, Dad, I did. I let us both down. I'm sorry, Dad. I really am. I know I don't have the right to ask you for a favor, but do you think you could ever forgive me for what I did?"

Marc was in tears at this point, eyes closed, seated in my big, black, La-Z-Boy. He told me that he silently responded to Matthew and that of course, he forgave him. That was the easy part. The hard part was accepting the fact that he would never again see Matthew. That was the heartbreaking realization. The men continued to process this conversation silently in the quiet of Marc's imagination. They decided that Matthew would be in charge of their two late dogs, Duke, the German Shepherd, and Connie, the Retriever, the other two great losses that had devastated both men. Marc imagined that Matthew would be waiting at the entry of a place called the "Rainbow Bridge" (I had never heard of the poem at the time), where animals go to wait for their loved ones when their time on Earth is over.

Marc was delighted to think that he would be reunited with Duke, Connie, and especially Matthew once again, upon his passing. In fact, he was able to put Matthew in a place in his mind where he would finally experience some peace. The way he conceived of it, Matthew was no longer suffering, he was reconnected to the dogs, and Marc would be reunited with all three of them at some future point. He, like Joe in the previous story, was still beset with a host of other issues to contend with, including marital and financial challenges, but Matthew was settled. He described our imagery experience as "that thing we did," and to this day will still say, "When we did that thing, I put Matthew on the Rainbow Bridge with Duke and Connie. I'm okay with that. I'll see them all again someday… And I've never felt an ounce of guilt since that thing we did."

Sacred Hearts

I like telling Marc's story whenever it appears to be relevant. One such opportunity was at a meeting of a group called "Sacred Hearts" in a nearby town. The only way to gain entry to such a meeting is to have suffered the death of a child at any point in life, from a miscarriage all the way to the death of a sixty-three-year-old son from a massive heart attack. The meetings begin with every member telling the story of their child's death until the room is thick with enough sadness to suffocate all the hope in the room...followed by a silence. When it is my turn, I realize that the speaker is supposed to offer the audience some semblance of peace after their tragedies. Never before had I felt such an intimidating responsibility. Parts of me wanted to feign sickness and bolt for the exit.

Of course, I didn't run. Instead, I chose to explain that their sadness was commensurate with their losses—the greater the love, the greater the sadness. And that holding onto the sadness was a way to hold onto the loved one. I also told them that the goal as I understood it was to hold onto the beautiful memories, stories, etc. provided by the loved one while accepting that they were gone now and would not be returning to Planet Earth. And then I told them about Marc's story and his imaginary meeting with Matthew and the dogs. I reminded them that Marc's guilt was his way to keep Matthew around. and that when Marc released them to the Rainbow Bridge, his guilt was no longer necessary.

And then two beautiful and affirming things happened to me: First, I received a standing ovation for the first and only time in a career chock full of speaking engagements and flattering responses. Secondly, I received the following in the mail, several days later:

Dear Dr. Cortman:

Please accept my sincere thanks for taking time out of your busy schedule to speak at our Sacred Hearts meeting. I want you to know that I found great comfort and wisdom in your words. I lost my son, Derek, in September 2008 to an accidental drug overdose. He had just turned eighteen, and he died in his own bed in my home on my watch. I have been suffocating in guilt. I am nowhere near ready to let myself off the hook for this, but after hearing you speak, I think I better understand why I need that guilt.

We do things because at some level there's a payoff. At this stage, beating myself up with guilt is preferable, thank you very much, compared to accepting the loss. And maybe that simple understanding will someday lead me to a better place than I am right now.

I truly believe you are a gifted healer and I thank you so much for sharing that with our group.

Sincerely,

Nan

Reframing and releasing have a complicated, intertwined relationship. At some times, releasing the pain in the past is sufficient for healing, while at other times, it may feel like there is a barrier to releasing. Reframing your thoughts, beliefs, feelings, and behaviors may need to occur before releasing. Thought and beliefs like, "I should have or could have" often are a barrier to releasing and accepting, as they breed feelings of guilt. The next chapter on reframing will explain why these feelings and beliefs need to be reframed.

Questions for Comprehension

—

What are the three best ideas that you gleaned from this chapter?

_____

_____

_____

_____

_____

What type of action do you believe is necessary to help actualize these ideas?

_____

_____

_____

_____

_____

How did you execute your plan?

_____

_____

_____

_____

_____

What is the result of your efforts?

_____

_____

_____

_____

_____

Chapter Seven

Reframe: Reclaim Your Life

"They say time will heal the pain, but it just goes on forever."

—38 Special

REFRAME

Okay, I get it. Things have been very heavy for you thus far, reading about molestation, rape, dying children, and gross-you-out combat scenes. But what if the worst thing in your life is a broken heart and a crumbled romance? What if your pain in the past is about the one that got away? Trauma is trauma. Everything I've written up to this point applies to your emotional hurt, whether it was a ten or a one on the trauma scale. Obviously, the more horrific the event, the more impact it's likely to have. Nonetheless, even more common, less catastrophic traumas can have a huge impact on your life, as the following example illustrates.

Nate is that guy who never had much "game" with women. Ladies described him as a truly great guy, and they loved him to pieces, but only as a friend. As a result, he lived his adult years "perpetually trapped in the friend zone."

But there is one woman, Angela, he likes to talk about, even now, fourteen years after she ended their "fling"—it was never anything more than a friendship and a drunken kiss one evening that took her by surprise. For Nate, this was the woman of his dreams, the one he should have married. Something went wrong, he believes, and he blew his best opportunity to be happy.

It's remarkable how sad he becomes when thinking about Angela and the children they never had together. Given that they had no more than three dates and no sexual relationship, nor any committed partnership, how does this sadness persist so powerfully in Nate's mind?

All behavior is purposeful and goal-oriented, and you do nothing without a purpose or a goal. Stated another way, everything you do meets a need, and everything you keep meets some perceived need, or you wouldn't keep it. Take a minute to go look in your closet and see if you can donate five articles of clothing to charity. Can you do seven? Ten? What are you basing your decision upon? Probably one very important criterion: you will keep all the clothes you believe you will wear again and discard the ones you think you won't. It's that simple. But it's true about your emotions as well. You hold on to things you need emotionally to help to define your life as you have.[46]

Nate, for instance, had the most joyous, rapturous couple of weeks in his entire life while sharing those few dates with Angela. He has experienced nothing before or since then that approximates the feelings he felt for her.

As I've emphasized, everything you do is about trying to improve, control, or manipulate your feelings. Nate is holding on to Angela in a desperate effort to maintain hope of again experiencing those feelings as in the time of life when he was happiest. Ironically, holding onto the memory of Angela—they are not in touch—does not afford him those rapturous feelings and hasn't since the breakup. Instead, thoughts of Angela now provide nothing but sadness and self-deprecation.

Mr. Avoidance, At It Again.

So why keep *those* feelings? It's simple, actually. To let go of those feelings is to let go of Angela, and to let go of Angela is to give up the possibility of feeling those rapturous, happy feelings again. Remember Mr. Avoidance? Nate is avoiding releasing Angela because keeping her on a lofty pedestal is superior to feeling lonely, defeated, and rejected. Maintaining the Angela fantasy prevents Nate from feeling his worst feelings. Nate is not going to say goodbye to Angela until he meets someone else who "makes [him] feel that way" again.

Mr. Avoidance can have especially deleterious effects on the ability or opportunity to reframe your thinking. Without possessing the opportunity to adjust your thinking in some way, these beliefs solidify over time. Because Nate had not spoken about his relationship with Angela (or lack thereof) with someone, he didn't give himself the chance for someone in his life to help him come to the awareness that he and Angela did not, in fact, have a romantic relationship (as you'll remember in the Express chapter, expression of feelings ideally should be shared with someone else). The consequence: he had placed Angela on a pedestal, and she wasn't going to be removed from the pedestal until he remembered, felt, and finally expressed his feelings to another person before releasing them.

Imagine seeing a concrete truck with its ever-rolling cylinder of concrete. The cylinder must continue to rotate at all times to prevent the concrete in the truck from solidifying and hardening. Mr. Avoidance stops the cylinder from rotating, and because of this, whatever it is that you are telling yourself about the pain in the past becomes solidified and is believed by you, the sufferer. And it becomes your reality. If you believe something to be true, it is true to your nervous system. Try to convince a Flat Earth Society member that the Earth is round, or try to convince a staunch Republican or Democrat to switch political parties. Regardless of the validity or strength of your arguments, if another person *believes*, your efforts are likely to be futile. Mr. Avoidance prevents the other person from having the opportunity of altering that belief.

Here's the real potential harm that can be done if Mr. Avoidance is allowed to operate: whatever it is that you, the trauma sufferer, believe (regardless of its validity or invalidity) will become your reality, and you may become stuck there. In the following stories, you'll hear about how people become stuck in their thinking and how that prevents them from reframing and healing. Becoming stuck and avoiding are the ingredients needed to fuel the fires of guilt, depression, anxiety, shame, or any negative emotion. And as you'll read, those fires can burn indefinitely if the pain is never expressed, reframed, and released.

How to Reframe

Nate's story isn't unique. Throughout this book, you have read how people will desperately hang onto things like alcohol, guilt, and resentment to avoid letting go of loved ones. To let go, you must not only say goodbye, but you must also reframe your pain in the past.

To reframe, you must first become aware of where you have become stuck in the first place. In the first session with clients, I usually ask them to communicate what happened in the past that has hurt them. After they've expressed their pain, I can gain insight into their thinking and what has prevented them from healing. I can see where they have become stuck. Once they've identified their stuck place, they can then reframe that particular belief.

What does it means to "reframe" something? Putting a new frame on an old picture creates a brand-new look by altering the appearance of the picture. Similarly, putting a new frame on a painful experience, trauma, or loss is necessary to release the power of the hold that this experience has over you. In each of the following stories, I'll lay out both where the individual got stuck and how the Reframe is done to help unstick the client.

COGNITIVE BEHAVIORAL THERAPY TO THE RESCUE

Martin Seligman, who is truly a giant of modern psychology and an expert on positive psychology, uses the term "explanatory style."[47] According to Seligman, how you explain the world to yourself is more important than what is really happening. His research demonstrates, for instance, that depressed people explain their reality with more self-blame, negativity, and pessimism about the future than non-depressed people. Conversely, he has discovered optimistic thinking is associated with many positive outcomes, including with cancer, pregnancy, and surgeries, in addition to improved mental and emotional health.[47] So, where, how, and when would you inject optimism in your explanations to yourself regarding a traumatic event? When is at any time from the moment that trauma occurs to now. Thinking well about your trauma—reframing—is listed as the fifth step of the Fritz, but in practice, it's a component of every step. Even during the trauma, it is vital to self-instruct in a healthy, problem-solving, rational way, as you will see below.

Let's take another look at the two types of categories alluded to earlier, the traumatized and the grief-stricken. We understand that these categories often overlap, as in Jim's case from chapter one—we will return to Jim in a bit.

The traumatized individual, you will recall, needs to somehow digest the horror of the experience by remembering, feeling, expressing, and then deciding to release the incident(s). But to finish the story, you will need to explain the story to yourself in a different and healthier manner than you have to this point.

Dan, Continued

Let's return to Dan, the Vietnam veteran who lost his friend in combat (see Chapter 4), literally inches away from him in a rice paddy. The self-instructions in the situation included the following: *Stay down and in control. Be calm, Dan. I'm just going to wait until there's a break in the shooting and drag him out of here. I can get him back to the medics, and he'll be okay. Just follow the orders!*

From what Dan told me, it appears that his thinking and reacting in the moment was similar to the above and largely responsible for his survival. He didn't stand up angrily and charge the enemy for killing his friend. And during this worst-case scenario, his training took over, and his thinking was about nothing other than survival.

The trouble for Dan and for so many others is how they explain the trauma to themselves afterwards (which is where he became stuck). Let's peek into some of those cognitions and Dan's explanation of that trauma:

> *I don't know why he had to die, it should have been me. I don't deserve to live—what have I done with my life to make a difference? It was my fault anyway. What kind of a friend am I when I allowed him to die in front of me like an animal? Those f***ing gooks deserve to die for killing him, and I wish I had killed more of them, at least that would have been something. Instead, I shot and missed repeatedly. If I had done my job well, he'd probably be alive. I don't deserve to be alive, let alone happy.*

Note the emergence of guilt (survivor's guilt) in Dan's thinking. Dan became stuck in self-blame, self-punishment, and an unwillingness to accept that his friend had died. Dan's cognitions help illuminate where he had become stuck. Beliefs like "It was my fault, I shot and missed, if only I had done better" perpetuated the guilt and kept him trapped in the past. Again, it is here that Mr. Avoidance helped to solidify these beliefs. Maybe if Dan had talked about his horrible tragedy with a close family member they could've helped him see that his friend's death was, indeed, not Dan's fault. But as stated earlier, Vietnam veterans as a group did not talk about their experiences. Granted, maybe it wouldn't have mattered if Dan had talked with someone else about it. Keeping the guilt helped Dan to feel powerful (I could have saved him), rather than powerless (There are untold casualties in war). Also, as long as Dan remained stuck in self-flagellation (guilt), he didn't have to say goodbye to his friend. Stay focused on the guilt and you'll never have to grieve your losses. Maybe Dan simply did not want to give up the guilt, because at that point, accepting what had happened (that his friend was dead) would be his only option. Mr. Avoidance (not expressing) prevents that opportunity from even happening. If Dan had talked about this experience earlier in his life, he might have been able to reframe and release it then, instead of forty years after the fact.

Once Dan identified the self-blame, self-punishment, and unwillingness to accept reality as the place he had become stuck, Dan could reframe his combat experience as if he were suddenly possessed by the spirit of the healthiest person in the world (a wonderful technique, you should try it).

The Vietnam War was not my fault. I joined because I support this country. I did not cause that battle, nor did I give the orders to go through this rice paddy. I did not order anyone to shoot at him. I simply followed protocol as I was expected to do, I did not deviate from it one bit. In fact, I was no more to blame than the poor guy who shot my friend, and he, too, was following orders. People die in wars, thousands of people died in this war. My friend was only one of them. I was fortunate enough to survive. It is up to me now to live the life I still have and find meaning in my losses and in having participated in a futile war like Vietnam. I'm physically healthy and capable of living a productive life. But I need to first say goodbye to the losses in my life, including both people and my innocence.

Expect to have thousands of thoughts regarding the trauma you experienced and your part in it. But to reframe that trauma in a healthy way is to think about it in a realistic problem-solving fashion. Realistically, Dan was not responsible for his friend's death or the deaths of more than 50,000 American soldiers in that war. The responsibility and guilt that Dan felt didn't belong to him, but for many years, Dan assumed the responsibility for his friend's death, and by so doing, blocked the grieving process. He never had to grieve the loss or even accept that he had been "used as pawn by his government in a meaningless war." To accept those realities removes the barrier of guilt and allows Dan to grieve those losses. Then he can choose to say goodbye to what is gone and hello to the responsibility of living a meaningful, productive life. If he continues to hang on to the guilt, he never has to make his life count for anything, because bad people (as Dan believed he was) aren't expected to live meaningful, productive lives. Be aware, though, this this is just one step—as important as it is to reframe your trauma, you must also remember, feel, express, and release it as well.

Tamika's Story

Like Dan, Tamika suffered a horrible trauma (see Chapter 4) and feared that she would never live to tell about it. Recall that she was abducted and held against her will, raped, and threatened until she managed to escape. Tamika also needed to reframe her "three days of hell" after feeling, expressing, and releasing (evicting) her perpetrator from her head with the goodbye letter.

For Tamika, the reframe became necessary after the abduction, because like Dan, she was remarkably composed and rational during her three-day abduction. She remembered telling herself survival-oriented statements like: *Stay calm. Don't oppose or incite him. There will be a chance to escape, and I will take that chance when it's time. In the meantime, don't give him any reason to hurt you. (During rape scenes, she told herself:) Go somewhere else in your mind. He is doing that, and it'll all be over soon. (And after the fact, she reminded herself:) If you get pregnant, you will have an abortion, just survive. You can and you will escape at the first opportunity.*

Despite this healthy, problem-solving thinking, Tamika suffered greatly during and after her abduction. Like Dan, she reexperienced her three days of trauma very frequently. (Recall that intrusive recollection of the event is one of the most prominent symptoms of PTSD, including frightening nightmares and spontaneous recalling of images, sensations, and feelings of the trauma.3) But as much as she had in common with Dan regarding his trauma, there were also some significant differences. Tamika's life was not dominated by survivor's guilt. In fact, she didn't feel guilty at all. If anything, she was righteously indignant that she didn't deserve the set of experiences that made up her trauma.

For Tamika, the emotions that so dominated her life (in which she had become stuck) were fear and rage. The fear she experienced consisted of feeling that "the world was unsafe now" because she had been abducted and tortured for three days and that this ugly experience was now part of her reality and life story and would never go away. Her reluctance to accept that this had happened to her essentially created another "part" of her that wasn't fully integrated into her consciousness. It was as if she were saying someone else had been abducted. (Tamika did not suffer from Dissociative Identify Disorder, though a fractured self can catalyze this disorder, which was previously known as Multiple Personality Disorder, and which I'll discuss later.)

Despite having distanced part of herself, Tamika felt rage toward the perpetrator, and she had become trapped in that anger. Why? Because forgiving and releasing him *felt like* condoning what happened, and she couldn't do that. Again, all behavior is purposeful, and staying angry at him constantly reminded her that what had happened to her was not okay.[46] Obviously, nothing about kidnapping and rape is okay, but Tamika's perpetual anger served to keep the stress response switch on (see Chapter 1). Mark Twain said it best: "Anger is an acid that can do more harm to the vessel in which it is stored than to anything on which it is poured."[24]

The goodbye letter was designed to help Tamika move out of the traumatic scene and release the images and the control that the perpetrator had over her mind. She needed to express that rage and release it, because hating him would only ensure his continued dominance in her mind and her life. If that meant that he got away with it, Tamika would need to rethink and reframe that too. We explored her religious roots to discover a thought that brought some comfort. "Vengeance is mine; I will repay, saith the Lord." (Romans 12:19, King James Version) And it was just as imperative in her recovery for Tamika to reprocess and reframe the world around her. Just as it had once been an idyllic place to live, it had become a treacherous place of imminent danger, scary people, and potential bondage.

Reframing for Tamika (which was partly encapsulated in her actual goodbye letter) would contain thoughts, attitudes, and beliefs like the following:

> *What happened to me was a very unusual experience. It is not likely to happen again. I will be more cautious as a result, but not hypervigilant (overly cautious) or paranoid. I will continue to live my life as a confident and happy young woman. I will not hate that man, because hating him only guarantees that he will continue to own me. I dismiss intrusive thoughts of him and will walk him to the door of my mind and re-release him. He has no place in my head anymore. I can find meaning in suffering; a lot of great people have. I will use the experience to learn more compassion for others, more patience,*

and more mercy. I will pray that God uses me to help others as a result of what I've been through. I will learn appropriate boundaries with people to use in all of my relationships. I will no longer live in fear! It is time now to put away the trauma.

Again, reframing the event allows you, Dan, Tamika—or anyone—to rethink the meaning of the trauma(s) and weave the experience into the greater fabric that is your life. As Syd and Suzanne Simon[26] have taught, it is no longer the central piece of your life, just one thing that happened to you in your life.

REFRAMING THE GRIEF-STRICKEN

Reframing is also necessary if your pain in the past is related to grief. You have read how Marc was able to alter his self-explanation regarding Matthew's death, but let's look at where he became stuck in the first place and how the reframe helped him heal. Marc did what every parent who has an addicted child does—everything he could. After Mark expressed his pain to me, I agreed that Marc had indeed, done everything right, and thus, when he asked me "What else could I have done?" I replied "Nothing!" Marc became trapped in the belief that *If I do everything right, I should be able to change the outcome.* The "just world" belief assumes that good things happen to good people and bad things happen to bad people. So when Marc's son Matthew died, it was a stark contrast to this belief system. Marc was trapped in a "How could this happen to me, when I did everything right?" belief that prevented him from accepting his son's death and letting go of the guilt and anguish. His reframe took place during the guided imagery and has never wavered since that exercise. When he thinks of Matthew now, he claims:

"I know my son did the best he could, but he could never get past the problem he had with drugs (opioids). His twenties were one long battle with drugs, which honestly made us all quite miserable, especially Matthew. I realize there wasn't anything I could do to save him, I tried everything. I guess it's like they taught me that time I went to the twelve-step meeting, I didn't cause it, couldn't control it, and couldn't cure it. I was as powerless over Matthew as he was over the drugs. So now, I tell myself that we all did the best we could, even Matt, but sometimes that's just how things end up. I'm okay with it, I just keep seeing him smiling, happy to be on that Rainbow Bridge with the dogs licking him and fetching sticks in the water.

I don't think of his life as a waste anymore, I see it more as a struggle that finally came to an end... If I think of God's part, I think of God as merciful, not punitive. I don't think that God 'took Matt,' I see it as God allowing Matthew to escape his suffering and move on to a better place. My wife struggles more with Matt's death than I do, but she never did that thing we did (guided imagery) where we put Matthew on the bridge. That was so real to me that I haven't questioned where he is or whether he is okay. Since that day, I'm all good with that. You know it does help to know that his brothers are okay, because I realize that all three boys were different even though we raised them the same. You know what else is helpful to me? The boys who are doing well in life are still here. And the one who struggled and suffered has moved on to a better place. I'm quite able to live with that, and rather than being guilty like I used to be, I've learned to be grateful instead."

Joe's Struggle to Reframe

Joe, father of Joey, also needed to reframe his son's death, especially to make sense as to why a father should have to bury a son and how to give meaning to Joey's life and premature death. At first, of course, he kept returning to his "life is good" toast as if that had triggered the heavens to swallow Joey up. But it wasn't so much self-blame and self-criticism that consumed Joe, it was trying to make sense of the tragedy, as if there was some concealed meaning as to why kids can be taken from their parents. Joe, like Marc, was stuck in what felt like unfairness; that while Joe and Joey were both, by every measure of the concept, good people, still Joey had died. But in addition to being stuck in unfairness, Joe had become stuck because he couldn't figure out a meaning or a purpose for his son's death, and without this meaning, Joe found it difficult to let go and accept what had happened.

Reframing for Joe was about trusting that things happen in life that make no sense to anyone. The loss of his son was truly senseless, and it wouldn't help Joe to believe that God wanted Joey or had a purpose to call him home. What made more sense to him was that Joey died because he fell off a mountain. Nothing more, nothing less. He could accept that, because it prevented him from agonizing about why God didn't reach out a hand and catch or save Joey. God didn't work that way, Joe recognized. Things happen. And yes, bad things do happen to good people, much like in Harold Kushner's book *When Bad Things Happen to Good People*.[22] It was not because God didn't love Joey or his parents, and it was not because of anything that Joe or Joey had done that deserved punishment. Joe had to accept that uncertainty and that no logic existed that explained his son's death, other than that it was an accident. With that in mind, Joe still needed purpose or reason to get involved in life again. Guided imagery was a reminder of several things for Joe, and he was quick to spell them out for me:

Maybe the most powerful realization for me was that Joey is not only still alive, but he is truly immersed in love. He is happy, alive and well, not broken or defeated. I can't feel bad for him, I know he's fine. I do feel bad for his siblings, for myself at times, but especially *for his mother and his children, as we all miss him terribly. But no more pity for Joey. He died doing what he loved and continues to live with purpose in the beyond, or at least that's how I have construed it in my mind. As far as missing him, I know that's normal. I still miss my father, and that's been, s**t, twenty-seven years now. But it's not a crushing depression, just a sadness that reminds me of how much I loved someone who is no longer here... It's funny, but just having Joey ask me to step up and be there for his family helps to provide me with a purpose that wasn't there before the imagery. Rather than believing that all is lost, now that my Joey is dead, I know that I am charged with a mission to be the best grandfather I can be to his kids. I don't know, it just feels like a purpose that I cannot ignore. What I like best about it is the sense that instead of feeling powerless as I did, I now feel challenged with a type of mission where I need to step in for my dear son, because he can't do it for himself. I find myself feeling grateful to God for having important things to do that honor God and honor Joey.*

Joe's reframe consists of the new-found ability to accept that in an imperfect world, parents can and often do lose children through no fault of their own. Secondly, Joey died because he fell thousands of feet to the ground, *not* because God is spiteful, Joey was bad, or his parents were being punished for some reason. I asked Joe, a Catholic Christian, to consider the scripture where Jesus' disciples asked, "And his disciples asked him, saying, Master, who did sin, this man, or his parents, that he was born blind?" Jesus responded, "Neither hath this man sinned, nor his parents: but that the works of God should be made manifest in him." (John 9:2–3)

Again, it is imperative to reframe the tragedy by finding meaning in Joey's death. Part of that meaning became Joe's need to be a better father than he had ever been before and an even more loving husband, as well as a newfound passion to be a male role model and father figure for his grandchildren.

The reframe was a challenge to honor God and Joey by living his life in pursuit of being worthy of that calling.

What about the Atheist?

I can hear some of you asking: What about the atheist? Will these techniques work effectively if there is no God, and no world beyond this one? Rochelle was a woman in her late seventies who was accomplished, humorous, loving, and very straightforward. An ethnically Jewish woman with no belief in a higher power, she lost Rachel, her forty-five-year-old daughter to cancer. Rachel was, at least in Rochelle's eyes, the best person on the planet. She described her as a brilliant, kind, salt of the earth kind of child, who made every life she touched better. Losing her was the single toughest thing Rochelle had to face in almost eight decades of life.

Naturally, I told her about guided imagery and the need to gain some closure, but Rochelle refused to use this technique to allow Rachel to say that she was alive and happy. According to Rochelle, "When you die, you die, and there is no more."

Nevertheless, imagery was indeed helpful, in that both women were able to say things that Rochelle needed to say and hear (from Rachel). And despite the lack of potential for a later meeting date, Rochelle was afforded an opportunity to hear Rachel say, *"Even though I am gone, mom, and I'm not returning, I still want you to be happy and I want you to continue living a good life without me."* Divine intervention or a belief in an afterlife is not required to trust that the person you loved who is no longer here still wants you, the bereaved, to be happy as they did in life.

Despite the belief that she was saying goodbye to her daughter forever, Rochelle benefited from this action. She reframed Rachel's passing by emphasizing that her daughter had enjoyed a well-lived and worthwhile life. She also recognized that no one would have wanted Rachel to continue living in pain as her body was being consumed by cancer. For Rochelle, the adage that it was far better for her to have loved and lost Rachel than to never have loved her at all was certainly true, and this helped her to say goodbye. From all indications, Rochelle's treatment proved to be very healing, as she returned to therapy shortly thereafter when her husband died to work toward releasing him as well.

What about Nate?

Nate, our love-sick martyr carrying an eternal cross for Angela, was stuck in a fantasy due to an unwillingness to accept reality (avoidance), or perhaps an avoidance of painful emotions like disappointment, rejection, and loneliness. What can he do to reframe his loss? Essentially, he needs to tell himself the truth:

> *My fantasy version of Angela, is just that, a fantasy. She never thought of us as more than friends, so the "lovers" relationship existed only in my mind and is no more a reciprocal relationship than the one I have with Michelle Pfeiffer or Cindy Crawford. So why do I keep hanging on to Angela? Because I like the high of thinking we had something special, when really, I was infatuated but had only found a new friend, nothing more. I can release her and put energy into meeting other women through friends and online dating and be more realistic in my pursuits in terms of age and level of attraction. Everyone tells me that a beautiful woman on the inside is a far better choice than a beauty queen, anyway. Most importantly, I want to be with someone who loves me for me, someone with whom I share values in common values, and someone who is truly my best friend. Maybe it's time to write a goodbye to Angela and thank her for the many life lessons I've allowed her to teach me.*

The Purpose of the Reframe

Earlier in the book, I spoke about the stress response and how detrimental it can be if left in the "on" position. These reframes move your brain from the intensely stressful "it's horrible" position to the less stressful "it's okay." By believing it's okay, you can turn off the stress response. Once the stress response is finally off, you can release the pain in the past and live in the present with purpose and meaning. By turning off the stress response, you can finally refill your emotional energy and use that energy in more effective ways.

You probably were aware that the individuals profiled in this chapter had little to no responsibility for the traumas that threatened to destroy their lives. However, this is not always the case. Sometimes the one holding onto the pain is also the one who has culpability in having caused the pain. In the next chapter we will explore how to reframe if you carry some responsibility for what happened.

Questions for Comprehension

—

What are the three best ideas that you gleaned from this chapter?

_____

_____

_____

_____

_____

What type of action do you believe is necessary to help actualize these ideas?

_____

_____

_____

_____

_____

How did you execute your plan?

_____

_____

_____

_____

_____

What is the result of your efforts?

_____

_____

_____

_____

_____

Chapter Eight

Moral injury: What If You Really Are Guilty?

•

"You're only as sick as your secrets."

—AA Big Book

MORAL INJURY: WHAT IF YOU REALLY ARE GUILTY?

You have now read several stories of how innocent, loving parents often assume toxic guilt when their children die in accidents. You now understand how and why you may remain in guilt because it protects you against the need to accept reality and say goodbye to your loved one. Removing the protective guilt allows you to deal with the real issue—the incredible sadness from the loss of that loved one. And as you are able say goodbye to the beloved, you can permanently release the guilt. Once again, please note that the guilt was misplaced anyway. It was undeserved, because you did nothing wrong in the first place. Your loved one died through no fault of your own.

But what if there really was some culpability on your part? What if you did contribute to or cause someone's death? Cheat someone or steal from them? Commit infidelity? Neglect or abuse your children? In other words, what if you really did do something wrong that caused a deleterious outcome for someone? Perhaps needless to say, making mistakes is a significant part of the human journey. Mistakes and poor choices infiltrate even the healthiest and most successful of lives. Without making terrible mistakes, we would never learn the great lessons of life on Earth.

THE CONCEPT OF MORAL INJURY

As you might imagine, psychologists treat many, many people who have been violated by others, and you have read many of these accounts already. But sometimes, the person we see *is* the culprit—the one who has perpetrated the pain. For the purposes of this chapter, let's focus on several true stories of people causing or contributing to the death of others. Sometimes these others were people they knew and loved very much; sometimes the victims were complete strangers to them. I will also include different types of perpetrators, including the now recovered alcoholic or abusive parents, who left many an invisible scar on now resentful adult children. I will share the real-life process and outcome for each of these people and then some psychological and religious input on self-forgiveness when it really was your fault. Please allow me to share the backstory first and then the healing process later in the chapter.

Ruth's Story

Ruth was on vacation, enjoying her wonderful family, when suddenly she took a very hard fall, sustaining a back and neck injury in the beginning of a series of disasters. The major foundations of her life (family relationships, health, financial security, spirituality) began to fall like dominos as one disaster after another ensued, culminating in the following tragedy:

In an effort to treat her significant physical and emotional pain, Ruth relied on medications. Her regimen included a mix of chemicals that not only made her pain tolerable but created a debilitating drowsiness that put Ruth in bed for hours each day—something that she had never experienced before. One day, Ruth and her husband Ira were babysitting Jessie, their three-year-old granddaughter. Ruth was suffering more than usual and called to Ira, who was cleaning the swimming pool at the time. He heard her call, came upstairs to see what she needed, and inadvertently left the gate to the pool unlocked. Jesse found that opening and drowned.

Losing a three-year-old is a devastating blow for even the healthiest of families. But to lose a child due to a simple mistake like failing to latch a gate (because you were responding to the call of an ailing wife) is even more crippling. Imagine having to tell your daughter what had happened. Ironically, perhaps, it was Ruth and not Ira who absorbed the lion's share of the guilt for Jessie's death. Piggybacked on top of the loss of her health, her job, and her financial stability, now she felt a combination of guilt for having called for Ira (and for being bedbound and nonfunctioning) and a resentment toward him for having left the latch unlocked. Marital difficulties ensued, and by the time I met Ruth, she was suicidal, depressed, and in a state of self-loathing. But was it necessary for her to assume responsibility for Jesse's death to say goodbye to her? We'll return to Ruth later in the chapter.

Holly's Story

Holly was thirty-two years old when I met her, although I would imagine she was still being "carded" if she wanted to order an adult beverage, given her youthful appearance. She presented with depression that was not responding to medication, and as a result, she was referred to me by her primary care physician for treatment.

As is often the case, Holly was depressed because of her outlook on the world. Essentially, she was very self-deprecating in her thinking and saw her life as futile. To use her words, "There's just nothing to look forward to anymore." This last statement, especially with the word "anymore," allowed me to peek under the hood, so to speak, to decipher what had sucked the hope out of young Holly's life. What I learned I will never forget, because it's just one more time I had to admit that this could very well have happened to me.

Holly had a brother, Tyler, seven years her junior. She adored Tyler as older siblings often do, especially when the difference in age disallows the development of a sibling rivalry. Instead, Holly conceived of herself as a junior mother to Tyler; he was her little boy. But one day when she was nineteen, she took her brother out for the day. They stopped first at a large department store, where Tyler temporarily became lost. Holly was horrified that something terrible had *almost* happened to Tyler on her watch! She would not be able to live with herself if she allowed something to happen to her "Baby Tyler." Two hours later, Holly made an error in judgment behind the wheel of her vehicle, and twelve-year-old Tyler was killed by an approaching truck. Holly walked away physically unscathed but emotionally ruined for the foreseeable future. Tyler's life had been snuffed out before he could even finish middle school, and it was all her fault. What could anyone say or do to help Holly overcome depression twelve years later, when she was still burdened by the realization that "I killed my favorite person in the world"? To me, it was little wonder that the antidepressants were ineffective—they don't have a pill to remove the guilt of killing your little brother. Again, I will return to Holly's story later in this chapter.

Elizabeth's Story

Elizabeth is the grandmother every kid loves. Thoughtful, attentive, affirming, generous—she scores straight A's across the board. But as awesome as Elizabeth is now as "grandma," that's how poor she was as a mother. Elizabeth was a "raging alcoholic" by her own words and "a horrible drunk" in the words of her oldest living son, Samuel. Samuel had an older sister, Joy, who fell victim to a drug overdose in her late adolescence. Both Samuel and Elizabeth blame the latter for Joy's death, especially because Elizabeth was not much of a force in her children's upbringing. She was too drunk to be a parent.

Elizabeth wasn't always a drinker. Her alcohol abuse began shortly after her husband Ted died in a freak construction accident when the kids were nine and five. Raising two young children was a very difficult task for a young and freshly widowed homemaker. Elizabeth struggled with the unending demands of being the primary caregiver. When Ted died, there was a settlement, not enough to retire on, but enough for Elizabeth to avoid the prospect of having to work, at least for a while. Besides, her friends reminded her it was better for her kids if she stayed home with them, as they were already devastated by the loss of one parent. Losing her also was inconceivable, yet lose her they did, at least figuratively. Elizabeth hid her sadness and fear in an ever-present bottle of Absolut. She liked that vodka didn't make her sick, and from her standpoint, it was undetectable to the kids because there wasn't a strong scent of alcohol.

What there was instead was a self-absorbed, "self-piteous mother" with a lightning quick rage and a bitterness that penetrated any and all of her children's defenses. There were legions of broken promises, embarrassing bouts of holiday drunkenness, and the prospects of a passed-out mother on the family couch with the TV blaring and nothing cooking, at the end of a school day. Not exactly Donna Reed. The kids would talk about their two lives—the one "before Dad died" and the "disaster that followed" with Mom at the helm, each day looking forward to school and sleep, as they were the places that mom's ugly behavior could not penetrate, or at least not usually. There were times she showed up at school, half in the bag, with a lunch box or homework assignment in hand, something inadvertently left at home. The children were left with the ensuing public humiliation and the fear that the other kids would tease about "your mother, the drunk." The kids, as is often the case, traveled in their different directions: Joy turned to drugs, while Samuel became a basketball fanatic.

Elizabeth continued to drink heavily, but when seventeen-year-old Joy's accidental overdose resulted in death, things deteriorated rapidly. Elizabeth indulged in self-pity—life had taken two of her family members through no fault of her own. She was pulled over for two DUIs in six months. The second time prompted the judge to take decisive action—she was deprived of a driver's license, placed in jail for one month, and given probation for a year, along with court-ordered treatment (following a substance abuse evaluation). Elizabeth complied with and successfully completed the latter and has been sober for the past eleven years due to a "religious" commitment to the AA program and its twelve steps and traditions. She is almost 180 degrees different in her attitudes and behaviors from where she was in her self-described race to self-destruction.

The grandparent role was much easier for Elizabeth, given that she was sober and could always return the kids to Samuel and his wife. Elizabeth's newfound commitment to honesty and sobriety brought her to the fourth step in AA (a fearless moral inventory). She was able to remove her protective glasses in favor of a more realistic perspective on her role in Joy's death. She concluded that she had abandoned her children when they needed her the most. She believes that had she responded to Ted's death as a hands-on, loving, and reassuring mother instead of disappearing into a bottle, Joy might still be alive today.

Suicide was another option Elizabeth contemplated, especially when realizing that she had failed in the most important role she had ever played in her life—parenting the children to whom she had given birth, the people she loved the most. No matter what she did, Joy was gone, and to Elizabeth, escaping from the horrible guilt she felt through suicide appeared, at least at the time, to be a better option than always feeling like a failure.

But working with two people, one in her past (her AA sponsor, a retired minister) and one much more recent ally (me), afforded her a new perspective, which included the capacity and willingness to reengage with her family as a grandmother and as a mother to young adult children. But more on that later...

Mr. Avoidance Rears His Shameful Head Again

Moral injury complicates the healing process and makes it more difficult to traverse alone. Lacking moral injury, the grief-stricken may still become stuck in guilt—it hampers the grieving process and prevents people from letting go. In most of the stories up until this point, after finally confronting the trauma or the death, the clients usually accept that they have little to no responsibility for what happened to them or the deceased. Guilt usually results from thinking that you "should have, could have...known that this bad thing could be stopped, prevented, avoided, [or] changed" and that in the end what *you did was bad*. Without moral injury, guilt stems from a **perceived** violation of your own moral code, not bad behavior.[46]

Shame, which is what the clients in this chapter are experiencing, is the belief that *you are bad*. Elizabeth, Holly, and Ruth have become stuck in shame, the belief that they are bad or immoral for letting Jessie drown, or accidentally killing Tyler in a car accident, or neglecting children.

Think of it this way. If you've raised kids, you know that they will eat some "forbidden" cookies. When asked, "Did you eat those cookies I told you not to eat?", they will say no, despite the smeared chocolate evidence on their impish faces. When do children tell these lies? When they feel shame! A researcher named Lawrence Kohlberg developed a model to explain moral development.[48] He noted that young children are basically dichotomous: when they act bad, they feel bad, and acting good makes them feel good. In adulthood, you tend to hide the things that you are ashamed of. You typically don't hear adults bragging about the third slice of cake they ate, public flatulence, missing their daughter's piano recital, or relapsing on alcohol.

Enter Mr. Avoidance. When you are responsible for the abuse, neglect, death, torment, or negative feelings of another, the normal response is shame. Imagine the shame that the Ruths, Hollys, and Elizabeths of the world feel. You can appreciate how and why they *actively* avoid talking about these traumas. The importance that shame plays in the development and maintenance of trauma-related symptoms cannot be understated. Humans like to be liked. Shame is the belief that you are bad. People *do not* like talking about anything that they are ashamed of. This is where the steps of remember, feel, and express come into play heavily. You must remove your shame from the closet and expose it to the light of day by expressing it. Then and only then is healing even a possibility. Remember, shame, like traumatic memories, will never heal when hidden in the recesses of your mind.

The quote in the beginning of the chapter alludes to this thought process. "You're only as sick as your secrets;" in other words, the shamefulness of alcohol abuse must be brought to the surface and exposed for all to see. Once it is exposed, then you have a choice to make regarding what to do with that shame. I'll share two biblical stories to help illustrate this point.

GION AND MORAL INJURY

◇

biblical, nondenominational Christianity—was an
eptualizing the Fritz. The biblical message, at least as I
understand it, is that God loved sinful man enough to forgive him for all
transgressions (King James Version). Old Testament forgiveness required
a sacrifice of an animal to demonstrate contrition, including confession
(admitting to the sinful behavior), repentance (doing a 180 degree turn
away from sinful behavior), and making amends (trying to compensate
somehow for the damages done). If God found the sacrifice and acts of
contrition acceptable, the sins would be forgiven (i.e., let go, as if they had
never happened).

With the New Testament came the story of Jesus, reported as the only
begotten son of God, sinless in his own right, yet a willing sacrifice for all
mankind. No longer was it necessary to sacrifice an animal, as Jesus was
the Lamb of God, who in his sacrifice and subsequent resurrection took
away the sins of the world.

In this same New Testament, there are several stories of men and forgiveness.
Tax collectors Matthew and Zacchaeus were guilty of bilking the public of
money for their own personal gain. Upon meeting Jesus, these two gentlemen
not only confessed (admitted) to their crimes, they also repented from them
(stopped) and made amends by compensating their victims four times as
much money as they had stolen in an effort to reconcile the error of their
ways. (Luke 19:1–10, King James Version.)

But there are two outstanding stories in the New Testament of gentlemen
who mucked things up, big time. These gentlemen have unique stories and
yet had remarkably different responses to their mistakes.

Judas Iscariot

Let's begin with the consensus bad guy of the New Testament, Judas Iscariot. As many of you know, Judas was one of the twelve disciples of Jesus. On the evening of the "Last Supper," Jesus reportedly prophesized that, "One of you will betray me" and then proceeded to toss a hunk of bread on Judas' plate. (Matthew 26:21, King James Version.) Judas abruptly left the room, and according to the scriptures, he sold Jesus for thirty pieces of silver. And then, after evidently realizing the mistake he had made in betraying his master, Judas chose to hang himself.

Saul of Tarsus

Saul of Tarsus was yet another New Testament story of a guy who believed he had made huge mistakes. A Jewish Rabbi and a man of great influence, Saul was reportedly incensed by the new religious movement of the day, wherein followers of Jesus were proclaiming that they had seen their Lord risen from the dead. But Saul was having none of it—he reportedly was arresting these Christian zealots and jailing or killing them as fast as he could.

One day, as the story goes, Saul was heading to a town called Damascus when he was blinded by a great light. He also heard a voice asking, "Saul, why are you persecuting me?"

Saul responded, "Who are you?"

"It's Jesus, whom you are persecuting," said the voice, and the rest of the story is well known within Christianity. (Acts 9:3-9 King James Version.) Saul changed his name to Paul and proceeded to become the most prolific Christian missionary and PR guy of all time. Despite having been imprisoned himself, shipwrecked, and stoned nearly to death with rocks, Paul had a simple message he needed everybody to hear: "I am the chief of sinners, and yet I am forgiven." The good news (gospel) is this: "You, too, can have your slate cleaned by a loving God through Christ His Son, and I intend to share this news with all people in the world." And so, Paul wrote no fewer than thirteen Epistles (letters), which are included in the New Testament. Today, of course, he is known as Saint Paul, one of the most influential religious leaders of all time.

So, what's my point? These were two men who had both screwed up mightily, at least in their own eyes. One of the men could not bear to face his guilt and shame and took his own life. The other man believed he was forgiven (and was therefore forgivable) and spent his days traveling the (known) world proclaiming the good news that if I can be forgiven, you can, too, because I am worse than you.

How does that translate 2000 years later into the lives of people who have committed wrong during a lifetime? Several important ideas can be gleaned from these two stories (even if religion isn't for you). For one, there is a choice. You can stay stuck in the worst thing you've ever done. Whether you've stolen, committed infidelity, physically assaulted someone, neglected a loved one, or bullied a disabled kid, whatever it was, you may also choose self-forgiveness, à la Saul of Tarsus, and make the world a better place with your redemptive efforts.

APOLOGIES CAN GO A LONG WAY TOWARD FORGIVENESS

Dr. Aaron Lazare, a University of Massachusetts psychiatrist, wrote a landmark book, "On Apology," explaining the importance of apologies in promoting healing, from global atrocities to personal affronts.[49] He demonstrated that effective apologies require complete ownership of responsibility for the behavior by the offending party(ies). Of course, stating "I'm sorry" or "I was wrong" is often insufficient. Expressing remorse is also helpful, as is an explanation of the faulty thinking that existed at the time of the offense. Other potentially helpful aspects of an apology may include commitments that these behaviors will never happen again: "I am sober now and will never drive inebriated again," or especially attempts at making amends: "Included in this letter is a check for $____ to pay for the repair of your fence."

So, for those of you keeping score, a proper apology requires four things.

1. Complete ownership of whatever it is that you are responsible for, "no 'buts' or excuses allowed."

2. A sincere and genuine, "I'm sorry."

3. Repentance; discontinue the behavior that got you in trouble in the first place; do a 180-degree turn away from the offensive behavior.

4. Making amends, which includes repairing what is broken, fixing the problem, etc.

Without these four elements, an apology typically falls short of its mark. Think about the spouse who repeatedly says, "I'm sorry, how many times do I have to say it!!" Well, without taking ownership of the misbehavior first, saying "I'm sorry" falls on deaf ears. The cheating spouse who apologizes for infidelity but then continues to cheat (not discontinuing the bad behavior) nullifies the apology. Apologies that are demonstrably sincere and accompanied by a change in behavior, however, are vital if one hopes to gain forgiveness from others.

But is self-forgiveness as simple as being sorry and turning away from your transgressions? Let's return to the people you read about earlier in this chapter to learn just how they managed to make peace with the personal horrors that ended up destroying the lives of others and thus ruining their own lives.

HEALING WHEN WE ARE AT FAULT

Ruth

Ruth is the devastated grandmother of little Jessie, who drowned in her pool. As you know, guilt is used as insulation against saying goodbye to a loved one, especially a three-year-old child. And shame keeps this horrible tragedy hidden in the closet, away from the reality of what occurred. My approach to her horror story was to help her remember, feel, and express her sadness, guilt, and shame with me at great length. Her anguish was commensurate with the degree of her trauma. What can anyone say to assuage the terrible loss of a child, especially in the aforementioned manner? I continued to encourage her to express her emotions, with the hope of some semblance of release or at least a degree of acceptance of her loss.

Desperate to help her, I tried a Hail Mary pass; I suggested a guided imagery exercise where Ruth, a Jewish woman who believed in both a loving God and the promise of an afterlife, had the opportunity to meet one more time with her granddaughter. Again, I spoke for Jessica but included an angelic being who could communicate on behalf of the child. Again, I made it clear that death was the result of an accident, that God was punishing neither Ruth nor Ira and certainly not the child. No one needed to be holding grudges or blaming anyone, but God would use this accident to bring his people closer to him and would provide a blessing for all who trusted in him. Further, I spoke to Ruth about accepting the challenge of trusting that Jessie was with God and believing that she would be happy and that she was now in a place where she would never suffer any more pain or strife. She belonged to her Creator and was literally in the most peaceful of places. Once again, the message was to never forget Jessie, but not to use her memory to cast a shadow of sadness upon the family's future. "Remember me as someone who brought you joy and not sorrow," were the words spoken from Jessie's angelic representative; "Please go and live in peace."

The imagery was extremely emotional, as Ruth emptied half a box of Kleenex. I wanted to believe that was a sign of compliance with the procedure (as it almost always is) and an indication that she had been able to successfully visualize the meeting with Jessie.

What followed surprised me. Ruth said not a word for over three months, no appointments, no comments about the procedure, until one day she sent a card requesting that I perform a guided imagery process with her son, the young uncle of the deceased. With that written request was the following note:

> *"Guided imagery made the crying stop. It worked! I'm able to function and not have a breakdown. I feel really different! It worked—I can't believe it. Thank you so much. I cried all day (previously)—it's just different. I was a hard nut to crack; for you to get me to that point was amazing. Amazing!"*

And within the next year and a half, Ruth had something else to share: Her daughter had another beautiful baby girl. Much like the story of Judas and Saul, this gift from God's bounty provided her with an opportunity to either dive in and love again or withdraw for self-protection. What if something happened to the new baby? But after completing the guided imagery, Ruth approached this as an opportunity to love again; an opportunity not to forget about Jessie, but to love Jessie and her new granddaughter. From all indications, healing and self-forgiveness had taken place.

Holly

Let's return to Holly, the young lady who lived through the incredible misfortune of driving her car out into the intersection where her brother was crushed by an oncoming truck. Stuck in perpetual shame, she was the perpetrator who had killed Tyler! Try to imagine what that must have felt like for her, to have killed the person you cherish most in this world. For me, there was no hesitation regarding the treatment plan. I knew I would request that Holly participate in a guided imagery exercise as soon as (A) she felt that she was safe with me and that I understood her pain and how that was so inextricably linked to her depression, and (B) she knew that she was ready to meet with Tyler again to finally bring some closure to his awful death.

After working to ensure that Holly was adequately relaxed and capable of visualizing the meeting between herself and Tyler, I allowed her to create the site where she and Tyler would meet. I instructed that she was allowed to hug and kiss him when she first laid eyes on him. After a long and tearful embrace, she released him and envisioned Tyler glowing. Still a handsome cherub, he had that same glow that Charlton Heston wore as Moses in "The Ten Commandments" after meeting God. In the guided imagery session, Tyler took charge of the meeting at first, allowing Holly to understand that his visit was by special permission, and that while he could not say a lot about where he was and what he was doing, he was very happy, busy, and surrounded by love. He told her that he knew that she loved him—she was an awesome big sister, and he felt adored by her, not bullied—and that he loved her just as much. He knew his death was an accident, nothing more, nothing less. She was no more a bad person than he was for falling off his bike or skateboard. It was an accident! He needed her to know that he wanted something from her. Tyler requested:

"I know that you have been hurting terribly since the day I died. Please understand that I never hurt—one moment I was in the car, and the next moment I was in a new body, in a place so beautiful, I can't even describe it to you. I am not sad, I am not lonely, and

most importantly, I am not angry at you. I am happy and busy, and everyone is loving!

I want to ask you to trust that I am very well and want for you to be well, too, Holly. You need to forgive yourself for the accident, as I forgive you. Listen, I can tell you this: One day, you will be here with me, but don't ask me when. In the meantime, you have a life to live. Holly, it doesn't feel good to me to think that I ruined your life. I want to believe that you are happy and living a meaningful life. Don't get me wrong, sis, I want you to remember me, but as someone who brought you joy, not sorrow. I want you to get strength from my memory, not feel sick to your stomach every time you think of me. I want you to let me be here happily while you live the rest of your life happily as well, until it's your time to come here. I will plan a big celebration for you when you arrive, but I'm guessing that won't be for a long time. But know that it's okay to stop crying for me—I think it's about time that you are happy again too. Oh, and one more thing: Tell mom I love her also and that there are no curfews here! Thank you again, big sister, for being as awesome as you are. Now go and live your life in joy—all is good!!!"

A box of tissues and an embrace later, our exercise was completed—no longer unfinished business. The imagery technique was real to Holly, so real that she wanted only to believe all aspects of her visit with Tyler.

During the next session, she made two extremely validating comments; first, "I am truly at peace with Tyler. I tried several times, but I can't even go into a dark place about it. It's better." Secondly, she said, "My mom wants to come in and do what we did. After all, it was her son."

Although Holly may have indeed made an error in judgment while driving that morning, it is a forgivable mistake. Shame is a powerful poison that will erode people's happiness, but forgiveness is an effective antidote. The guided imagery provided Holly with the opportunity to be forgiven by her deceased brother, Tyler. And with that forgiveness, Holly could stop punishing herself with depression, guilt, and shame at the mere thought of her brother. Instead, she could live happily in Tyler's honor, per his request.

Elizabeth's Healing

Healing and forgiveness can start in various ways and take different paths to absolution. Following the death of her husband, Elizabeth began excessive alcohol use, the death of her daughter accelerated it, and it all culminated in her DUI conviction, where she was court-mandated to go to treatment. For Elizabeth, her "rock bottom" had been reached when she spent a month in jail. She then decided to comply with the treatment and chose a path toward healing that began with treatment. While her decision to stop drinking was influenced by the criminal conviction, ultimately, she had accepted that she had a problem with alcohol and decided to attend her first ever Alcoholics Anonymous (AA) meeting. Her apology began with repentance (doing a 180 degree turn away from the behavior) when she discontinued drinking alcohol following her second DUI.

Elizabeth began the healing process while in jail. The thirty-day sentence had "sobered [her] up" through the very uncomfortable withdrawal period. But while there, she began to accept that she had "a real problem" with alcohol, and after getting out of jail, she complied with her probation, including abstinence and participation in AA. Elizabeth, like so many people in recovery, noted that "attending the AA meetings is helpful, but the real change in sobriety occurred when I found my sponsor and started working the twelve steps (of AA)." Enter the retired minister, a woman who Elizabeth explained had her own twenty-year history of alcohol abuse and now sponsored newcomers in AA. The woman told Elizabeth that volunteering as a sponsor was, for her, "living the twelve steps."

Elizabeth, who had been sober for eleven years by the time I met her, told me that she had "bought in" early on and attended daily meetings. Within months, she began working the twelve steps with her sponsor. Over the course of a year, she had remained substance free, completed probation, continued AA voluntarily, and completed seven of the twelve steps of AA. As you readers in recovery may know, there are similar themes present between the four steps of an apology outlined above and several of the steps of AA.

Repentance—doing a 180 degree turn away from the bad behavior—is, of course, the very crux of AA's purpose, which is to maintain sobriety. Once again, an apology is meaningless if the bad behavior persists. The first step of apologizing, as outlined above (taking total responsibility), is step four in AA (taking a fearless moral inventory). For Elizabeth, this included admitting to God, herself, and her sponsor that she had emotionally hurt, neglected (at times), and embarrassed her two children, Joy and Samuel. The final step of an effective apology listed above is identical to step nine of AA, which is to make amends directly, if possible. As a minister, her sponsor was able to use her own recovery and spiritual wisdom to help guide Elizabeth to successfully complete these steps, which included delivering a proper apology to her son, Samuel. She was able to share with Samuel, who hadn't been speaking to Elizabeth after the death of his sister Joy, her fearless moral inventory, which included the responsibility she'd had in his and Joy's difficult childhood.

She also, of course, apologized, and explained to him that she had been sober for a year. Elizabeth also made it clear to Samuel that her intentions to make amends had limitations, in that she could neither turn back time nor bring Joy back, but she could be the best grandmother on the planet. Recall that a proper apology can go a long way; Samuel took a leap of faith and began the process of reconciliation, and he allowed his mother the opportunity to be a grandmother. At first, he was tentative, but as she continued to earn his trust again, she was given more and more time with her grandchildren. Because of this process, Elizabeth now has a great relationship with her grandchildren.

I was the other helpful person Elizabeth met. While she was able to apologize to Samuel directly, she was unsure of what to do about Joy, because she felt Joy had paid the ultimate price. Her guilt and shame regarding Joy's death was still prevalent in her life. As a result, I recommended she write an apology/goodbye letter to Joy and read it at her headstone in the local cemetery. It read as follows.

Dear Joy,

This is long overdue, but I think I'm finally ready to apologize for letting you down, and hopefully, to let you go. Please let me explain: after your dad died, my world fell apart. It was never supposed to go down like this, your dad dying and leaving us behind to fend for ourselves. Granted, I know it wasn't his fault that he died, but the challenge of raising you and Samuel was mine alone after that. It was challenging, and I failed. I was too wrapped up in myself and my own grief. Dealing with losing your dad and raising two young kids was overwhelming for me, and instead of trying to get help, I was weak and turned to alcohol. No one "blamed" me for it at first, but it definitely got out of hand. I know I let you down because I was drinking all the time, and I think you suffered from that the most because you were the oldest. Seeing your mother drunk all the time no doubt influenced the young girl who became a drug addict herself. I turned to alcohol for support after your dad died, and I suppose that you turned to drugs because you didn't have support from your mother. I understand that now, and I am so sorry I wasn't there for you. I don't blame you for your drug addiction. Somehow, I hope you can forgive me for mine.

I have been sober now for eleven years, but I still feel at fault for your overdose. While I know that what happened to you might have happened regardless of my sobriety, I am working on forgiving myself and making amends to your niece and nephew. I know I wasn't the mother you needed, but I am working to be an unforgettable grandmother, and I hope that maybe that will be good enough. I love you and I miss you, and I'm looking forward to seeing you again when it's my time.

Love, Mom

Austin Wright

The final story in this chapter is about a young man who epitomizes what happens when you're feeling guilty because of the pain you've caused someone and how to cope with this trauma and move on with your life. I want to share this story in part because I observed it unfolding, and in part because it's inspiring to learn how Austin handled a situation that might have destroyed others. You'll hear directly from Austin how he came to terms with the tragedy he catalyzed and found the strength to lead a meaningful, productive life.

On April 2nd, 2007, twenty-one-year-old Austin Wright was in Gainesville, Florida, drinking and partying with his friends on the night of the NCAA national championship game. The University of Florida prevailed in the contest, defeating Ohio State '84–'75. Predictably, the city of Gainesville was alive with student celebration, with bars, clubs, and restaurants jammed with happy Gators. Austin was not a Gator, but both his parents and brother were. He had also attended nearby Santa Fe Community College, also in Gainesville. As far as he was concerned, this was his school, this was his team, and this was his celebration.

But then Austin made the worst mistake of his young life. He got behind the wheel of a car and ended up driving down a closed road and hitting a pedestrian, Lieutenant Corey Dahlem, forty-eight, of the Gainesville Police Department. The impact knocked Lt. Dahlem to the street, where he stuck his head on the rim of a parked vehicle and died instantly. Lieutenant Dahlem was a decorated police lieutenant, a husband, and the father of two children. From every indication, this was a fine human being who had made the world a better place. Austin came to see me wearing a somewhat stoic exterior, but was inwardly broken, scared, guilty, and ashamed. His parents were well-known in his hometown of Venice as impressive people, loving, responsible, and good-hearted. But they were now twice broken. Though they demonstrated genuine compassion for the Dahlem family, they hurt from the knowledge that their boy was going away for a long time.

At the sentencing, the courtroom included Lt. Dahlem's family, friends, and coworkers, all testifying about the man they had lost due to Austin's poor decision. The other half of the courtroom featured dozens of Wright supporters who had made the three-hour trek to Gainesville to support Austin and testify about what a fine young man he was, despite his disastrous mistake.

I testified on Austin's behalf, informing the court that this was indeed a man of "ego strength." He was wounded, but strong enough to be accountable for his mistake. He made no excuses and blamed only himself. He was remorseful, I stated, and possessed the capacity to learn from his mistake.

The judge possessed great leverage in his sentencing decision—he could choose a minimum sentence of say, three or four years, or a maximum sentence of thirty years, if he were so inclined. The judge knew that Austin was not a criminal and was a well-liked student in school who used his social and physical stature to take a stand for the bullied and the downtrodden. He was a good kid who had made a bad mistake. What was the judge to do to achieve justice? The answer was ten years in prison, eight and a half actually served—a statement that drunk driving was not to be tolerated, but Austin would have a second chance at life when his sentence was at last over.

Austin is a free man today, and he cherishes his freedom. I asked him if he would meet with me and allow me to tell his story in this book. Austin doesn't make plans easily—plans feel restrictive after being confined for so long—but he jumped at the opportunity to share his experience, because he wants to help as many people as possible. We met for lunch at a local restaurant.

I asked him some questions regarding his life after prison, his emotional well-being, and his re-assimilation into society. Mostly, I needed to know what he had done with his crime; how was he explaining it to himself at this juncture? Now that he was free, was he able to live his life without the emotional baggage of guilt, shame, and worthlessness?

What follows is an accurate paraphrasing of Austin's thoughts and feelings regarding his moral injury, recovery, and attempt at putting his life together in the healthiest manner possible.

"What do you do mentally with the fact that you killed Lieutenant Dahlem?"

"I have to move on. It hurts my heart when I think about him and his family, but I can't dwell on that if I want to be well. When I was in jail, a man (a cellmate) asked me if I believed in God. I said 'yes.' He asked if I had asked God for forgiveness, and I said 'yes.' He said, 'Then you have already been forgiven. Now it's a matter of forgiving yourself.' That helped me. I can't control if anyone else forgives me, I can only control my attitude and my behavior. For instance, I have decided I will never again allow alcohol to influence my decision-making. That will not happen again.

I know it's not about me anymore. That is, I don't have the capacity to change the past. If I could bring back Lt. Dahlem, I certainly would. But now my options are either to use my experiences to make a difference and help others, or to wallow in my own pain and shame and accomplish nothing. Essentially, those are my options. If my life is to have any purpose, I need to take the next fifty years to make a difference. Otherwise, the entire experience and the life lessons are wasted."

"How would you like to make a difference?"

"I can always become a better person. When I was first arrested, I was on a GPS monitor, so being a better person meant spending as much time with my family as possible. Now it means learning to better understand people. It really seems to help them when I can understand them, especially when I can relate to their pain, suffering, guilt, and fear. I also have learned to become more compassionate as a person. It all emerges from an improved understanding of myself, especially as the better I understand my own emotions, the better I can relate to and ultimately help others."

"How do you intend to help others? Do you have a formal plan, or is it more an informal plan to improve the world, one human at a time?"

"Actually, both. I think of myself as already helping everyone I can by being a caring and compassionate listener. But I'm now working fifty hours a week and attending college because finishing my degree is everything to me. At some point when I am capable, I'd like to devote more of my time and energy to helping ex-cons who are trying to land of their feet. I am actually thinking of buying a house and renting four small apartments to felons who are having a hard time with affordable rent. I have been there, I understand what

they're thinking. I don't know what else I will do, I only know that this is of central importance to my life. I have the chance to live my life from here, and I am grateful to have that gift. I'd like to convert that gratitude into action to help other people, especially former inmates. Does that make sense?"

"Did the notion of an 'eye for an eye' occur to you, and did you consider suicide at any point to even the score with the Dahlem family?"

"Even when I was at my personal rock bottom, suicide was never an option. First of all, I love life. I realized that there was so much I couldn't control in prison, but I did have control over my attitude and my choices. Besides, suicide never evens the score. It makes it worse. Now there's another loss, and my parents are even more devastated. No, that's not a good answer. I have learned to thank God every day for my life, and I've learned to cherish my family, my life, my God, and even me. It's important to not only forgive myself, but also to love myself. If I hate myself, then I cannot forgive me, I can only continue to make poor decisions. Because no good decisions are made from self-hatred."

"What would you tell your someone who found themselves unforgivable?"

"God can forgive all things, and so can you. If you can do it, you can forgive it. When it comes to your mind and your body, you are your own god. That means you always have choices. Again, if you can forgive yourself, then you are forgiven.

But remember, forgiving yourself is more than telling yourself to move on. Self-forgiveness is really about taking complete responsibility for my actions—it was nobody's fault but mine. And then, of course, self-

forgiveness requires changing my behavior. My self-forgiveness and apologies would be very empty if I repeated that behavior in some way. I must improve. My choice is to allow myself forgiveness. And then it's a matter of paying for the crime. On an earthly basis, I paid for my crime by doing my time. On a spiritual basis, I believe God offers forgiveness out of his own love for us. I have to believe that he loves and forgives me, so I can forgive myself."

As you might read in Austin's answers, his method of self-forgiveness harkens back to the Old Testament mentality of taking ownership (confession), changing the behavior (repentance), and cleaning up the mess as much as possible (making amends). This was corroborated in Dr. Lazare's work. No amount of apologizing or making amends will reverse his behavior on April 2nd, 2007, but Austin is aware of that. He also knows that he always has choices, self-contempt versus making a difference; Judas Iscariot versus Saint Paul. Austin chose the latter.

So, let's summarize what we've learned in this chapter: first of all, you are human. You will make thousands of mistakes throughout your lifetime. Most mistakes are benign, but some do significant damage to the lives of others, including emotional injury, bodily harm, and even death.

After making such a mistake, you have the option of running away, drowning in alcohol (or other substances), revising your core beliefs about yourself (e.g., "I am a loser and a failure, and always will be"), or facing the mistake head-on. Should you choose the latter, you must confess your mistake and take ownership of it. This mean repenting (seeking forgiveness), doing a 180-degree turn and not repeating the mistake (e.g., being clean and sober), and making amends where possible. Once done, you may then live the remainder of your life in gratitude by accepting forgiveness from God, others, and self, and using your time and energy to make the world a better place.

Questions for Comprehension

—

What are the three best ideas that you gleaned from this chapter?

_____

_____

_____

_____

_____

What type of action do you believe is necessary to help actualize these ideas?

_____

_____

_____

_____

_____

How did you execute your plan?

_____

_____

_____

_____

_____

What is the result of your efforts?

_____

_____

_____

_____

_____

Chapter Nine

Complex PTSD: When the Trauma Happened Again and Again

"Boy, you're gonna carry that weight, carry that weight a long time."

—The Beatles

WHEN YOUR PAIN IN THE PAST IS COMPLEX

◇

What do I mean by complex? In the simplest of terms, this involves ongoing and repetitive trauma. Having your father lose control and punch your mother is an ugly nightmare, to be sure. But your problems are worse when that situation repeats itself throughout your childhood. Repetitive or ongoing traumatic situations keep the stress response on and your nervous system on high alert for other potential threats. Exciting the stress response, you may remember, will take you from arousal (fight or flight) to resistance (continuing in high gear), then to exhaustion (breakdown begins), disease, and finally death. Old age, once again, is the accumulation of stress on the body.

So when children are exposed to ongoing or repetitive stressors, the consequences are far greater than dealing with a single trauma. Just as one rainstorm pales in comparisons to several consecutive years of extreme rainfall, so are many traumas more wearing and more difficult to treat than a single trauma. And now we have a term for the results of ongoing or repetitive trauma: Complex Post-Traumatic Stress Disorder (CPTSD).

What do we know about CPTSD? Quite a bit. Let's explore some of the differences between PTSD and CPTSD[51]:

PTSD	Complex PTSD
• Can result from a one-time event. • Often occurs in fully developed adults. • Affects emotions. Depression and anxiety are common. • Symptoms mostly specific to trauma. • Better prognosis for treatment.	• Results from accumulated traumas, often beginning in childhood. • Significantly affects social, psychiatric, cognitive, and biological development. • More severe emotionally disturbance, mistrust of others, defensiveness, and difficulties with interpersonal relationships common.

Essentially, it is PTSD on steroids. If you have experienced a single trauma, you'll need to process and digest your experiences through the Fritz (remember, feel, express, release, reframe). But if you've experienced multiple (ongoing or repetitive) traumas and have a likely diagnosis of CPTSD, you will need to utilize additional tools to effectively heal. While the Fritz can help you if you have CPTSD, you should also seek a properly trained trauma specialist to facilitate your healing. While working with a therapist, you may need to spend more time establishing rapport and trust, because trust is essential in rebuilding your broken life. Feeling safe with your therapist is also important, because your defensiveness was protective.

A therapist can help wean you off denial (denying the existence of problems and/or pain), minimization (downplaying the effects of said problems and/or pain), or dissociation (separating self from reality). You may need to take small steps before you will trust your therapist and yourself with the horrible memories you have pushed away from your conscious mind.

Once the Pandora's box of remembering is ajar, the memories are likely to surface—one at a time—until they are completed and depleted. This process of allowing the traumatic past to surface must be constructed upon a foundation of trust, connection, and safety. Things you have never told your spouse (or even yourself) you will now share with your therapist, much to your amazement. But to attempt to do so too soon may result in negative outcomes like early termination (dropping out of treatment) or feeling overwhelmed by the emotions of the memories and failing to cope (emotional dysregulation). Good therapy helps to establish trust, coping skills, and then a plan to bravely face the buried traumatic material (exposure to memories of all the traumatic events), which are all needed to complete the Fritz.

Ideally, it provides a therapeutic structure that helps you deal with all the intense memories and emotions at a tolerable pace. In reality, however, it's not always possible to control something that is like a lit stick of dynamite. Your memories can take on a life of their own, and when they appear, sometimes neither you nor your therapist are aware of what's about to happen.

SYMPTOMS OF COMPLEX PTSD

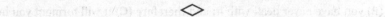

Symptoms of Complex PTSD can follow any ongoing traumatic experience, from childhood abuse to extended combat to a long-term abusive marriage. When trauma overwhelms the mind, there are many potential human reactions, depending on the age, personality type, coping style and skills, and level of family and community support, etc. Let's explore some of these reactions here.

Remember, if you're overwhelmed, you're prone to using various defense mechanisms that Freud theorized about, including denying that the trauma exists or believing that it isn't that bad, not remembering any part of it, or perhaps feeling that it happened to someone else (projection) or maybe that it happened to someone else that you created (multiple personality disorder, now known as Dissociative Identity Disorder, DID). So, it happened to other parts of you, but not you.

You can deal with your trauma by not dealing with it—yes, Mr. Avoidance again. And you may avoid it by abusing chemicals or compulsively doing something (working, social media, worrying, checking on things like door locks, praying, and even exercising). You may have your own way of avoiding it, or you may employ run-of-the-mill avoidance behaviors like listening to hours of new music, shopping until you and your net worth drop, binge-watching episodes of "Naked and Afraid," or some such preoccupation that separates you from your trauma.

But your body and nervous system is still aware of it. *The Body Keeps the Score*[52] is the title of a great book on trauma that communicates how emotional trauma manifests itself via physical symptoms. Your nervous system is aroused by a perceived threat (as you will remember by now) and remains in resistance, fighting the perceived stressors, until you later fall into exhaustion. You may also experience intrusive thoughts regarding your trauma which bring you back to the reality that (A) it did happen; (B) you have never dealt with it; and therefore (C) it will torment you in some manner until you do.

So I'd like to walk you through one case of a complex PTSD client, Leslie, who has been gracious enough to allow me to tell her story in uncomfortable (for her) detail. Her permission to allow me to write about her life demonstrates that she is happy with the progress that she made, and most of all, her hope that her story will inspire you to healing; she trusts that you'll recognize that if she could do it, then so can you.

Complex, ongoing trauma and the brokenness that abuse can wreak upon young children is treatable. By telling a very small part of Leslie's seven-year journey, I hope to convey that it's possible to rebound from even the most heinous of human experiences.

Leslie's Story

Leslie appeared to me to be a very depressed woman of almost fifty, a health care professional with an alternative life style and a profound sense that there was something wrong. Her depression symptoms contained the usual suspects: Dysphoria (low mood), anhedonia (loss of pleasure in the things she once enjoyed), apathy, sleep disturbance, negativity and pessimism surrounding the future, and a self-worth at the very lowest level. Besides all this, she hid her cocaine habit from everyone.

But Leslie had many other secrets that she kept not only from others, but also from herself. For one, she presented with a "psychic numbness;" she was not feeling much of anything and certainly nothing good. She knew there was something dark beneath her self-created anesthesia. It was as if she were learning to distance herself emotionally from the traumatic events from her past, although at the time, she didn't even know consciously that she had experienced any trauma, let alone a childhood chock full of horror.

There was another clue which served as a rather bizarre manifestation of a deeper problem than depression. Leslie was losing time in a form of amnesia. There would be chunks of time missing from her day, periods of hours that she simply couldn't account for or remember. Most people experiencing this problem would talk to their doctors and hope there were no neurological issues such as a tumor or traumatic brain injury. But neither Leslie nor I thought her brain was damaged—we both believed the depression, the numbness, and the lost time were part of something sinister lurking beneath the surface. She thought so because she sensed it. I thought so because of the many similar experiences I had previously had in my office where the symptom of lost time signaled that traumatic memories were about to surface.

Still, I suggested that Leslie be tested, and the neurologist confirmed that Leslie was asymptomatic: she had "a normal, healthy brain." But another symptom manifested itself: Leslie began experiencing flashes of being in another place and time. A childhood scene involving her father was appearing to her during her waking hours and then again in her dreams. I wasn't asking her to do any memory work, but rather was placing my emphasis on providing the safest atmosphere possible for Leslie to do whatever work she needed to do.

For instance, she was addressing her depression pharmacologically with antidepressants. I also worked with her using a cognitive behavioral approach, emphasizing that her thinking needed to be positive, problem-solving, and realistic, and that she should steer away from catastrophic thinking, self-deprecatory thoughts, and giving up. Behaviorally, I wanted her to do whatever was necessary to stop the cocaine. Ideally, I wanted her to trade it in for exercise, but she would not even consider giving up her occasional fixes with the white powder—we tend to hold onto what we think we need—and in the short term, Leslie believed she needed the cocaine.

Some clinicians would have made this a deal breaker and told her not to return until she was ready to give up her habit. I don't work that way. Recall in story that emerged with Rick, the man who was raped as a child by the magician, the healing work needed to be done first for him to give up the alcohol. This chronology is also true in other people I've treated who are suffering from co-occurring disorders such as PTSD and cocaine abuse, or depression and alcohol abuse. For them, some or all the trauma needed to be successfully extracted and healed to arrive at a place where the substance abuse could be addressed and stopped.

Again, I needed to be the safest person in the world for Leslie to get to where she needed to go. I set boundaries—she couldn't be high or drunk for our sessions, for instance. At the same time, I deferred to her in terms of timing—I recognized that Leslie wasn't going to do what she needed to until she was ready, not when I was ready. People like Leslie need to proceed at their own pace. Survivors of trauma, especially childhood abuse, often feel they control very little. Good therapy should not replicate the abusive relationship. Instead it should demonstrate that not all men are controlling and abusive (where the therapist is male) and that it is safe to partner with a therapist to proceed anywhere they need to go to heal from their traumatic childhood.

I told Leslie, "We will put on our hard hats with the flashlights on the top, hold hands, and venture forth into any dark rooms or caves that are necessary." But again, I had to earn that trust by demonstrating that I was a safe, experienced, and knowledgeable clinician, especially when it came to deal with unresolved traumas and pain in the past.

Leslie began experiencing fast-moving memories and further time lapses relatively quickly. The memories were horrible, involving a sick, perverse, biological father, who seemingly progressed in his pathology as Leslie's childhood went on. At first, her memories included scenes of incest, where her father would visit her bed in the middle of the night and drunkenly demand sexual services of a naïve, innocent preadolescent who was being introduced to a world that she was ill-prepared to survive, let alone thrive in.

Soon the memories were darker and even more painful to hear, involving scenes of human trafficking and multiple abusers. Eventually, Leslie began to remember scenes where she was taken to a farmland compound and introduced to people in a devil worshiping cult. She endured torture, abuse, and sacrificial ceremonies.

I had to walk a therapeutic tightrope. On one side, I was listening and believing my client, caring about her, and demonstrating genuine compassion for a type of suffering that was out of the realm of most human experiences. On the other side, I needed to find out what had taken place. I had to create a therapeutic distance between me and the horror stories, not me and Leslie. I could not feel her pain or fall victim to her terror. I had to be connected to her and compassionate about her suffering, but at the same time be therapeutically immune to the suffering. Failing to establish that curtain would expose me to the risk of experiencing what is called secondary PTSD or "compassion fatigue."[53]

And I was not alone in needing protection from Leslie's memories—Leslie herself couldn't deal with the abuse memories. For that reason, she created alternative or "alter" personalities to help her carry the memories, the emotions, and the behaviors that she couldn't handle alone.

ALTER PERSONALITIES

Can humans really create separate selves or alter personalities, or is that merely the stuff of Hollywood movies?

From my considerable experience with trauma sufferers, alter personalities are not only real, but not as rare as you might think. Although fascinating, the presence of alters is not typically a high drama action film. It is much more common for the bulk of alter personalities to be internal 'children' who are hidden from the trauma sufferer (and everyone else), which would also mean that they wouldn't often surface when adults were around. Their jobs are to protect the core person from the horrors of the trauma and to harbor the memories, feelings, and even functions that the core personality cannot contain.

Let's try an example: if you were relocating your home or office, you would need to move lots of stuff. Most of us are ill-equipped to do all of that packing, carrying, and cleaning by ourselves. It is too big a project and normally requires helpers, otherwise known as friends and acquaintances. Carrying a couch to the truck, for instance, which is probably almost impossible for you alone, is much more feasible with a friend's assistance. Multiplicity (alter personalities) is not much different.

The horrors of trauma, especially if they are frequent, can also be too much for you to carry alone, and so you employ a host of others, though less than consciously, to aid you in surviving when you might otherwise be drowning in the terrible abuse.

Once you realize how effective an alter personality can be and how easy they are to create, you can use one or more to handle all of the challenges in life that historically would fall on your shoulders. I have seen people create alters to deal exclusively with cult activities, to deal with unwanted sexual experiences, to perform professionally (for example, Florence Nightingale was an alter personality housed in the body of an RN), and even alters who specialize in house cleaning. Some contain the anger from the abuse, some carry suicidal ideation and a plan to end the suffering, and some may even side with the abusers and strive to please them. But virtually all of the alters contain memories of which the core person is unaware, along with the accompanying feelings.

For you to heal from having multiple personality disorder or dissociative identity disorder, you need to use the very same Fritz method of remembering each one of the memories (one at a time), feeling the specific feelings, expressing them to someone, and then releasing the horror in favor of a new perspective on the pain and suffering from the trauma. It's the same method that works for a single trauma, but now it has to be applied to several or many memories.

Of course, it is often the alter personality who tells the story and expresses the feelings, as the core person is unaware of the horror story until it is finally expressed. When an alter personality shares the story(ies) that it contains and appropriately expresses the accompanying emotions, the alter becomes much weaker, to the point of losing their power and becoming ready for integration.

Repeat the process of remembering, feeling, sharing and expressing, releasing emotions and integrating (blending or fusing) the alters back into the person they were at birth, the core person.

In other words, by applying the principles of the Fritz, even a severe condition like multiple personality disorder (DID) or complex PTSD is treatable and in many cases, curable. As mentioned in the introduction, I have treated numerous trauma survivors and more than two dozen multiple DID clients. Seventeen of the latter are now finished with treatment, and they have now integrated their alters into one person, the way they were born to be.

A little insight as to who develops multiple personality disorder and why: Lawson (2018) found that approximately 95 to 97 percent of individuals with DID report having experienced severe childhood sexual and physical abuse.[54] In my experience, 100 percent of my DID clients were repeatedly sexually abused. Many experienced other atrocities as well.

Leslie's Trio

Within the first several months, I was exposed to three of Leslie's more primary "alters," beginning with Rachel, the late adolescent female who served as an internal guide or an "inner self helper" to me. If there were harbingers of things to come or omens of things that Leslie wasn't prepared to know, Rachel would provide me with that information. More than just an informant, Rachel was also seductive—she did the sultry voice, crossed one leg over the other upon her arrival in the office, and referred to me as "blue eyes," not Dr. Cortman. The irony of Leslie's being a fifty-year-old, self-described "butch" lesbian wearing jeans and a T-shirt was not lost on me. But Rachel was an important component of Leslie, the way oxygen is an important yet not easily detectable part of water. And needless to say, the appropriate response to Rachel's seductions was exactly what you might expect—warmth, but with no need to respond to the seductive elements. And as a result, Leslie felt more safe and secure, as I wasn't looking to prey on her or take her up on her awkward invitations. In this way, therapeutic trust was increased by my continued professional behavior.

"Eric" was Leslie's six-year-old male alter, who watched me from the inside before emerging as my little friend and consistent visitor. For a couple of years, no session was complete without a guest appearance from Eric. He took part in so many memories because he seemed to have a propensity to deal with dark, confined spaces. For instance, Leslie's mother would often punish her by locking her in a trunk much like a hope chest, and Leslie would reportedly disappear into the chambers of her mind, only to be replaced by little Eric. Eric was very attracted to my collection of stuffed animals (all of them gifts from former clients, most of whom had graduated and were now completely integrated multiple personality clients). His favorite was a snowman he dubbed "Frosty." Eric would never need to announce his appearance; he would simply stand up from my very low couch, rush over to Frosty, and sit on the floor in the corner, rocking his frozen friend. He was completely oblivious to the fact that he resided in the body of a fifty-year-old woman with bad knees, someone who was not inclined to sit on the floor at any other times.

The third member of Leslie's trinity of prominent alters was Maria, the older and more stable of the group. Maria carried the bulk of the horrible content.

She was sweet and unimposing, essentially all business and protective of Leslie. It was not unusual for Maria to tell me a horrible memory and caution me that, "Leslie does not know anything about this memory—when she absorbs what I'm telling you, she will have a very difficult time."

Secrets from the Self

I would often listen in amazement that a human being could be sharing the most horrific of stories with me, yet also inform me that she herself did not (yet) know the story she was telling me and therefore had not been able to digest it. When employing the Fritz, you must remember (i.e., expose yourself to the trauma), but then feel, express, and release the toxic feelings before reframing. In cases like these, Maria and Eric would be remembering a trauma for Leslie and expressing that memory to me completely. Unfortunately, the emotions that accompanied these traumas were often left for Leslie to process. As a result, after particularly horrible and traumatic memories (and they were all horrible), Leslie was faced with calling upon whatever coping skills she had in her arsenal, whether healthy or unhealthy.

For instance, after remembering that her father had begun to sell her sexual services to his friends and cohorts after realizing that he could make a handsome profit from his daughter's innocence, Leslie not only spent her weekend drunk and high, but also took out a razor blade and carved bloody lines on her left calf, a behavior she shamefully admitted she had not resorted to in more than a year at that point.

Ms. Avoidance

She also spent her days between sessions calling upon her own version of Ms. Avoidance (not an alter) by for instance watching hours of mindless TV, sometimes after a cocaine binge. She found evidence (and later learned from Rachel) that Rachel had made a contact to engage in a threesome sexual tryst with a man and a younger woman; Leslie returned to find $300 and drugs on her hotel bed. While Leslie was perplexed and horrified, Rachel was thrilled to think that she could make money for selling Leslie's fifty-year-old body.

Leslie made many other efforts to avoid the acute pain of realizing that she had been forced to participate in rituals of a devil worshiping cult in the Midwest. She would take extra work shifts to keep herself too busy to feel. At other times, she would dog-sit loving animals that could appreciate her kindness without expecting anything in return.

Of course, the entire concept of creating alter personalities is by design another form of avoidance. Instead of facing your pain and the worst thing(s) that ever happened to you, you farm it out to self-created "selves." And this is what Leslie did, first as a brilliant method to survive an unsurvivable childhood, and then to deal with the memories when they began to surface decades later.

Denial, Dissociation, and the Devil

Other times there were attempts to block out the memories and deny that the events had happened. Leslie wanted to call herself crazy or psychotic, two things she wasn't, but maybe believing herself to be insane would be better than dealing with and feeling these horrible stories. Worse, there were periods of suicidal ideations. "What was my life worth, anyway?" she wandered. There were no kids and no partner, and she didn't believe that her career had amounted to anything.

> "So what's the point? If all my life is now is a roller-coaster ride through hell, why do I need to do this? And why do I have to remember every little detail? I already get it, I was abused in every possible way: physically, sexually, emotionally, spiritually. I was made to serve devil-worshiping men and carry the seed of the evil one. I had

to participate in rituals that professed devotion to Satan and watch as children were tortured and killed. And now I have to relive it and remember all of the details. Why? What did I do to deserve this life? Why don't I just kill myself and move out of this awful life? Isn't God supposed to be all-forgiving? Maybe he can forgive me if I say I've had enough of this life. Why must I continue living, Dr. Cortman?"

There is a therapeutic answer to her rant, and it goes something like this:

"I'm sorry you hurt so much. I hear your pain, Leslie, and it is so unfair that you've had to experience all this abuse. Thank you for trusting me with all of this. We will get through this, one memory at a time. This will eventually be finished, and then maybe, just maybe, you can tell your story to help others. I know you didn't deserve the abuse. This is not justice for bad things you may have done in this or another lifetime. Know that there are children out there starving to death through no fault of their own. This world isn't a fair or just place—but I do know a lot of people who have used their suffering and healing to make the world a better place. Maybe someday that will be you, also. I say we keep going one day at a time. Are you okay with that?"

Suicide Attempt

During the time I was treating her, Leslie intentionally overdosed on tranquilizers, antidepressants, and Bud Lights. Since she didn't make it to the grave or the hospital, I didn't hear about it until she emailed me and said that she'd survived her suicide attempt, convincing herself, of course, that she couldn't do anything right. I got her into my office that very same day and steered Leslie toward whatever unprocessed emotion had contributed to her suicide attempt. I also convinced her to agree to a "no suicide contract" (one that holds to this day). We also managed to uncover the specific feelings or "culprit" that had most influenced her decision. Leslie had remembered another experience where several men had sexually abused her simultaneously. But that wasn't the pain that had made her give up. She had dealt with that before. Here was the problem: when she remembered the story, not once had she seen herself rebel, fight, or protest. Was she therefore complicit with the abuse? Had she wanted to be raped? Was she nothing more than "Daddy's little whore"?

There was an easy answer. Let me recreate the dialog through which it emerged.

I asked, "What happened to you whenever you did rebel? Dad took that well, didn't he?"

"Well no, not exactly."

"Weren't you tortured every time, from being tied to the bed for over a week to being put in the hospital with broken arms, legs, and ribs (she had a photo of this; Dad had told the hospital staff she'd been mugged and beaten up), with whiskey poured on your burns, including in your private area? I'm not sure the whole rebellion thing worked out for you."

Impressively, that was all it required to dismiss the "I'm a whore" mindset and the concomitant suicidal ideation and behavior.

But Can You Really Believe Such Improbable Memories?

I'm not a psychological policeman. My job is not to find facts, report crimes, or bring people to justice. I am not a twenty-first century, self-styled cult-buster. My job is to help people heal from their pain in the past, and I've learned that they can do so regardless of the degree, intensity, or frequency of the horror. Unfortunately, that can only be done one terrible story at a time, until the closet of memories has been emptied and all of them digested successfully.

That said, one of the reasons I selected Leslie's story is the compelling corroboration that she found in her efforts to prove or disprove her memories: her mother confirmed the stories of abuse, offering at least two memorable explanations for her own behavior at the time, followed by a heartfelt apology and a year of sobriety before her death. Her mother's explanation: "If he was on you, he wasn't on me." In other words, it was a relief to be left alone. Secondly, "If I ever tried to leave him, we would have been brought back to the compound, tortured, and killed in front of the whole group. I may have been a bad mother, but I wasn't going to let that happen."

Leslie's older brother, Tim, a true hero of hers, had rescued Leslie more than once from her father's torture treatment. Tim also remembers that when he got a little older and was about 6 feet tall with 200 pounds of muscle on him and a favorite hobby of hunting, he warned his father, "You will never bring me to that place again, or I will kill you."

But the biggest clincher for Leslie was her return to the scene of the compound where the cult activity had taken place. Long since abandoned, the outdoor altar where all the human and animal sacrifices had happened was still erect amidst the forsaken grounds, a testament to her tortured childhood and a priceless source of validation that her memories were real and she was not crazy.

Moreover, recovery of repressed memory, a long debated issue in therapeutic circles, has been experienced time and again by dozens of my clients, comprising at least fifty people over thirty-two years. Invariably, the clients were normal, nonpsychotic adults who benefited from finally remembering what was at one time too painful to hold onto when it occurred. (For more reading on this, I suggest Lenore Terr's Unchained Memories: True Stories of Traumatic Memories, Lost and Found36.)

Back to Leslie

As the cult story progressed, the memories reached new levels of horrors as recollections emerged of adults willingly sacrificing their children to improve their standing in the cult, Leslie being sold to a man for an entire summer, and plans to make her a high priestess that were thwarted when she could not produce a child for the group to sacrifice.

She called upon her aforementioned trio of alters and several other personalities that played smaller parts in her recovery. She even had an alter named Avedon who cursed me, called me a "know-it-all bastard," and promised he would win in the end. He also took out his wrath on a stranger one night at a gay bar when he "picked up a wimpy guy, beat him up, and then hit him over the head with a beer bottle." This was all unbeknownst to Leslie, of course, until Rachel shared the story with me. But as alters are fueled by the emotions contained in the memories, Avedon was quieted and healed after a memory in which the sixteen-year-old boy in the group that Leslie had liked was killed for not whipping her as instructed. Leslie showed me a photograph of the two of them arm in arm together before he was killed.

Eric ended up collecting snowmen of his own until Leslie complained (while smiling), "I keep finding little snowmen all over my house, I don't know what I'll do with these if Eric ever integrates." Eric told his last story and said goodbye to us almost four full years to the day from when Leslie had begun therapy, leaving a big void in Leslie's heart and a house full of stuffed snowmen. Maria also finished her work two months after Eric did, but not before she helped Leslie process over 150 different memories from a nine- to ten-year period of her childhood.

Rachel made sure she was the very last alter to go, as if she were shutting the lights off and locking up. She felt responsible for ensuring that Leslie was not only finished with all of the years of her painful past, but also that she was prepared to take on life on her own going forward. Her last mission was to assist Leslie in recovering a relationship with her mother before tearfully saying farewell to her blue-eyed psychologist.

Leslie's mother's sobriety began three years into our treatment. Because of her healing, Leslie managed to forgive her mother, and Leslie was able to spend the best year of their relationship together with her mother before her mother died, leaving behind a very sad daughter who legitimately missed her "mommy" for the first time. Two years after her mother's death, Leslie is at peace with her many pains in the past and is functioning as an employed caregiver for dependent seniors.

I have chosen Leslie's story even though most of you will probably not have one past trauma like hers, let alone more than 150 of them. But because of her courage, her perseverance, and a plan of attack that afforded her the opportunity to remember, feel, express, and release her horrors, Leslie has reframed her complex trauma with a very positive picture for her life.

Questions for Comprehension

—

What are the three best ideas that you gleaned from this chapter?

_____

_____

_____

_____

_____

What type of action do you believe is necessary to help actualize these ideas?

_____

_____

_____

_____

_____

How did you execute your plan?

_____

_____

_____

_____

_____

What is the result of your efforts?

_____

_____

_____

_____

_____

Chapter Ten

Jim Meets Fritz

•

"Memories can be beautiful and yet, what's too painful to remember, we simply choose to forget."

—Barbara Streisand

PUTTING IT ALL TOGETHER

Remember: Tell the tale in detail.

Feel: No feel, no heal.

Express: Let the water flow.

Release: Release for peace.

Reframe: Reclaim your present life.

By now you should have a good grasp of the Fritz five-step process, but you may have questions about putting all the steps together to produce the outcome you desire. Since I've often talked about the steps individually in order to explain them clearly, you may be wondering how they all flow together. For that reason, I'd like to show you how Jim used the five steps to achieve the healing he desired.

Remember: Tell the Tale In Detail

Jim, like most people who have experienced trauma, tried both actively (by drinking) and passively (by excessive working) to forget what had happened to him. And why not? Who would want to remember the drowning of his two sons? He spoke of "trying to move on and forget," but of course, he could not.

Jim was overwhelmed by sadness, anger, guilt, shame, the intrusive recollections, the nightmares, and the pitying faces of those who felt sorry for him. It felt never-ending. To cope, he sometimes acted out by getting drunk and "racing the motorcycle" at 100 miles per hour. When asked about this, he replied, "I didn't care if I died." To Jim at the time, death was preferable to remembering.

Jim was pulled over by local police several times—the loud revving of the engine was sure to attract attention. But the police always drove him home or called his wife Ruth to get him because, "They couldn't send me to jail knowing what happened."

Other aspects of his life began to show cracks. Jim, who had been raised a Catholic, fell out of touch with his church. "How can I go to church when I'm angry at God? God took my two boys. I'm supposed to go to church and pray to an all-loving, all-powerful God who allowed my children to drown in front of me. I don't think so." Soon thereafter, their marriage, which had been very strong, hit a rough patch. The death of children can challenge even the best of marriages. Difficulties with communication, anger, guilt, and a general lack of emotional intimacy contributed to the strain on their marriage. Ruth sought individual counseling following the tragedy, while Jim suffered alone. Jim began to experience difficulties at work. He became short-tempered with customers and coworkers as well as overly cautious in his business ventures and had a propensity to "work [himself] half to death." Sadly, most of these habits continued throughout much of his remaining life.

Jim and Ruth eventually moved to Florida to retire. But with nothing to occupy his attention, Jim's mind wandered back to the pain in the past. He still worked part-time as a barber and "wished [he] could work more." But one afternoon while sharpening his razor, Jim looked up to see that a mother had brought in two blond-haired boys. "They looked just like my boys. I had to go sit in the back and cry." Part of him was hopeless and ready to accept that this was "the best" he would ever feel. But this was also what convinced him to try therapy again. That moment had been preceded by forty-four years of suffering and a rock-solid skepticism that nothing would ever change.

Remembering and Mr. Avoidance

Jim's problem with remembering wasn't that he couldn't remember, it was the opposite: he couldn't stop remembering. The daily memory intrusions and the nightly dreams were followed by guilt, shame, and relentless self-flagellation for "letting them down." Remembering wasn't necessarily the problem; Jim would argue that an inability to forget and move on was the problem. Our old friend Mr. Avoidance was running amok again.

Mr. Avoidance was at the helm in many of Jim's choices and operated in some obvious ways. For instance, while Ruth went to seek psychological treatment, Jim, despite encouragement from his wife's doctor, did not seek counseling because he "didn't want to talk about it." Jim did try psychiatric medications several times but noted no benefit. Instead, he preferred the comfort of Jack Daniels and Johnny Walker. If he drank until he blacked out, Jim didn't have nightmares; not a long-term solution, but it brought him temporary relief. Jim had always been a hard worker, but after losing his two boys, it was as if he could not stop working. Working excessively was

too real." The shame fueled Mr. Avoidance's power in Jim's life and even prevented Jim from becoming emotionally close with Michael, because his son was "better off not having a father than having a bad one." Guilt and shame never left Jim. They worked nonstop, twenty-four hours a day, 365 days a year to destroy any semblance of self-respect.

Though guilt and shame are arguably two of the worst emotions a person can feel, they were purposeful. When I asked Jim if he was aware of why he felt guilt and shame, he said, "No, I want to stop feeling this way, that's why I'm in your office." I explained to him that despite how horrible he felt, he was embracing them for a reason. There is always a payoff. In fact, guilt and shame were employed to avoid sadness. Guilt and shame needed to be reframed and released. Then he could feel the sadness, grieve the loss of his boys, accept having lost them, and finally let go.

Sadness, of course, is a natural and normal reaction to loss, and the loss of a child is the most profound of losses. But Jim was unwilling to experience sadness, because sadness requires acceptance. Feeling sad means that the tragedy actually happened and cannot be undone. To Jim, sadness meant that his sons were gone. The sadness, and Jim's inability or unwillingness to acknowledge it, supported by his use of the guilt and shame to help him avoid the sadness, eventually developed into what we call PTSD. Again, for Jim to heal, he had to remember, feel, and express in full detail what had happened.

EXPRESS: LET THE WATER FLOW

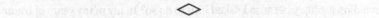

There are many different and effective ways to express emotion. I asked Jim to write a detailed account of what happened that day. If you remember the story at the beginning of the book, the ice skates had been early Christmas gifts for his sons. His boys falling through the ice and Jim diving under the ice to try to find them were among the details that Jim wrote about. I needed to know the whole story of what had happened that day. Knowing the whole context of what had happened provided me with the information I needed to help him reframe the trauma, remove the guilt and shame, and eventually say goodbye to his boys.

I asked Jim to *purposely* remember the worst day that ever happened to him for the first time in his life and write it out in detail and then tell me about it. Not surprisingly, Jim did not like this idea. He told me that he "can't and couldn't." He told me he was incapable of recalling these details for fear of "having a mental breakdown." I assured him, "If you're going to have a heart attack, it'd be best to have one at the hospital, and if you're going to have a breakdown, it would be best to have it at your psychologist's office." He laughed. I wondered if he would complete the writing assignment before our next session.

At 4 p.m. the next Friday, I walked out into the waiting room—no Jim. I proceeded to call him. He answered, gave a generic "I'm sick" excuse, and scheduled for the following week. My "Mr. Avoidance" alarm was ringing. He knew I expected him to complete the assignment. I suspected that he'd cancelled his appointment because he hadn't done it. Shame was operating again, and since he hadn't completed the assignment, he'd struggled with showing up that day to say so to me directly.

He did come in the next week. When I asked him if he had completed his homework assignment, he told me he had "tried but couldn't bring [himself] to do it." He had spent forty-plus years avoiding this, why would he stop avoiding it simply because I asked him to do so? In my many years of trauma treatment, clients often balk at the idea of *purposely* remembering the worst thing that ever happened to them. Jim and I then spent time exploring his difficulties completing this assignment, and I gently reminded him that this was in fact avoidance, and that avoidance was the culprit. After an hour of encouraging him and explaining that he'd tried his way, so he ought to try mine, I asked him, "Have I convinced you yet?" To which he replied, "I guess so, doc."

The next session, Jim returned with several pages detailing the exact events that transpired the day of the tragedy. I asked him to read what he had written aloud so that we could share it. He told me about the excitement of that day, sneaking away with the new ice skates, the sound of the cracking ice, the horror on his sons' faces, the paralyzing cold of the river, and the anguish of uncertainty. Local police from the county he lived in, police from neighboring counties, and hundreds of his friends and their families, along with local churches and their entire congregations, had all come and volunteered for the search party. For three days, they searched.

At this point, Jim had gone through about two-thirds of a box of tissues. Jim cried in my office like his boys had died yesterday. Though a great deal of sadness was evident, his primary emotions were guilt, because it "was [his] fault,"—and shame, "because [he] deserved misery." Though the guilt and shame were not ideal, through expressing his story to me, he and I became aware that these emotions were the barriers to the sadness and were blocking his completing the grieving process. The reframing step of the Fritz would need to be completed before he would be able to say goodbye to his boys.

REFRAME: RECLAIM YOUR PRESENT LIFE

One particular problem for people who have lived through trauma is their interpretation of events. Depending on the individual, reframing must occur before sadness can surface. Jim was one such individual. Self-blame, guilt, and shame became barriers to healing. Blaming oneself for events that befall your children is easy. Jim's story was full of "should haves" and "could haves." He believed that he should've been watching his boys more closely, even though they were only several yards away. He believed that they shouldn't have been outside playing, even though they had played outside safely hundreds of times before. He believed that he shouldn't "have been on that damn ice in the first place," even though they had played hockey there since the boys could walk. He believed he should have found them, even though he nearly drowned himself trying to do so. He believed he should have searched harder, even though he spent three straight days without sleep.

In forty-four years, he never questioned all the things that he "should have" done. As a result, all the blame belonged to him. Jim prided himself on being a good parent. In his mind, he had committed the ultimate sin of "letting" his children die. Jim's reason for existence was to provide a better life for his sons. And he'd let them die. He believed he was "evil, lazy, immoral, and destined for Hell as a result." Once this line of thinking began right after the accident occurred, it solidified because Jim didn't allow anyone to question these beliefs. This is how and why Mr. Avoidance can be devastating for the trauma sufferer. Reading all the things Jim "should have" done, it is easy to say, "Jim, you did everything that you could have." But Mr. Avoidance prevented that discussion from ever happening. Self-blame became a fixed belief.

When Jim finally expressed what happened, we were able to explore the entire context of the drowning. Then we went a step further to explore his relationship with his sons overall. After his sons fell through, about thirty seconds had passed before he was under the ice as well, looking for them.

We went on to talk about the "rule of threes" in a survival situation. An adult can survive for three minutes without air, three hours in extreme weather, three days without water, and three weeks without food. An adult who is underwater has three minutes to be saved and resuscitated before drowning. As children, his boys had even less time (due to smaller lung capacity). In ice-cold water, they had maybe two minutes at most (and even that is a generous estimation). Despite his heroism, Jim lost his boys that day. Nevertheless, Jim's belief that it "was [his] fault" was simply not true.

Jim went on to tell me about their relationship. He told me of fostering a love for motors and driving in his sons, envisioning that one day they would restore vehicles together. He built a small 50 cc bike from the ground up for them. His wife was not happy about that, but he and the boys "enjoyed the hell out of it." He spoke about the joy of wrestling on the floor of an evening well past their bedtimes. He told me that "even though they didn't have much money, the boys never wanted for anything." Jim and I spoke about how the boys had played outside hundreds of times before, how they had played on the river every winter, and how they were well-behaved, would come back when called, and were respectful of each other and adults.

Jim loved his boys and that his boys loved him as well. I told Jim, "There is no doubt in my mind that you did everything you realistically could have, and I believe that still, today, if you could trade your life for theirs, you would." He tearfully agreed. "And it is a fact that your boys are gone from this plane of existence; and while this is sad, it is also a fact that this was not your fault, not your responsibility, it was simply an accident." Jim, due to the influence of Mr. Avoidance, had never questioned whether it might not be his fault. His thought process of self-blame, guilt, and shame had solidified. Taken as a fact, his conclusion was never disputed.

In Jim's case, the important thing to remember is that reframing the event doesn't entail changing the event. Reframing means changing one's perception of what has occurred. For Jim, it meant aligning his perception with reality. Since Jim wasn't responsible for the accident, there was no one to blame. Moreover, since the accident was not his responsibility, the guilt and shame he was feeling didn't belong to him. And while removing the barriers of guilt and shame was helpful, the sadness was still there and needed to be released.

RELEASE: RELEASE FOR PEACE

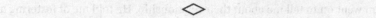

I saw Jim again two weeks later to ensure that the guilt and shame had stayed away and that only sadness was left. Releasing is one of the most challenging parts of treatment because it is about saying goodbye and accepting what has happened. After we talked about the options for taking this step, Jim agreed to write a letter to his two boys telling them that he loved and missed them and that he was saying goodbye for now. Jim appeared to again be reluctant, in the same way he had responded when I had asked him to purposely write about the tragedy; Mr. Avoidance was at work again. He and I processed these concerns, and with some encouragement, he agreed that letting go would be helpful. It didn't mean that he was forgetting about his boys. Again, we agreed that he would do this before our next session.

The next week, he again told me he hadn't completed the letter and that he just wasn't ready. We again spoke about how avoidance impedes healing, and I encouraged him, reminding him that this was the final step. "Not saying goodbye to your boys is mowing 90 percent of the lawn and then stopping, it's not putting the final piece in a puzzle, it's reading the whole book except the last chapter. Following this goodbye will be closure, peace of mind, and getting your life back." Again I asked, "Have I had convinced you?" and again he said, "I guess so, doc."

The following week, he came in with the letter completed; it was short and sweet, but it hit its mark.

Dear Kevin and Jim,

I don't know the words to say how much I miss you both and how much I love you both. I'm so sorry to you both. Not that I caused what happened, I know that now what happened wasn't my fault. I'm sorry that I haven't let you go and rest sooner. I am ready to do that now. I want to just have the happy memories of you without the sadness that followed, and I think I know how to do that now. So, I am saying goodbye to you for now. I am looking forward to seeing you again one day.

Love always,
Dad

As you can imagine, reading this aloud was highly emotional. Forty-four years of grief and sadness came rushing out when Jim finally said goodbye to his sons. We again worked through about half a box of tissues. I congratulated him for completing this task, and I asked him, "Do you feel like you've said goodbye?" He said, "Yes."

Following Up

I saw Jim at monthly intervals following that session. Having completed all five parts of the Fritz, Jim told me that his quality of life had improved greatly. He told me while he was at work, two young boys had come in. He was able to interact with them, joke with them, and laugh with them, all without the punishing guilt or sadness. Jim said he had been working to reestablish communication with some of his old friends, friends who were around when his boys passed. He told me that he had avoided people "who knew me at that time." Recently, however, he had reconnected and been able to "talk about my boys and the past without becoming a babbling mess."

His third son, Michael, noticed the changes, too. Michael told Jim that he "didn't really understand what was going on with you and mom when I was younger. All I knew is that I had two older brothers who weren't here anymore. But as I got older, I started to understand what happened." Jim told me that Michael had been "praying for me to get help for years." Jim said, "My wife says I'm much easier to deal with, which is the closest I'm going to get to a compliment. So you're her best friend now." Jim reported that he felt "unburdened," like a great weight was lifted off him. He noted that he has better focus and concentration and that he felt "like [he had] more mental space available."

Jim had let go of the pain in the past, and for the first time in a long time, he was able to really enjoy the moment and look forward to the future.

Thoughts on Jim's Story and the Fritz

As I noted at the start of the chapter, my goal here was to provide a single story from start to finish that demonstrates how the steps of the Fritz are put into action.

I've also told this story in order to illustrate how Mr. Avoidance will creep into the healing process at every possible opportunity. Be aware of and vigilant for Mr. Avoidance. In Jim's story, you see avoidance at every step of the process. When remembering, Jim tried to forget through excessive drinking, not seeking treatment (despite his wife's doctor's insistence that he should), and his motorcycle death wish. Jim avoided sadness through his use of guilt and shame. Sadness needed to be avoided because sadness was admitting that his boys were gone. He stopped communication and even moved away from the people who were aware of what had happened to his sons. Even with me, when I asked him to write about what happened, he became "sick" and pulled a no-show for his scheduled appointment.

By not reframing his thinking, he was able to avoid the entire context of what had happened (he had done everything in his power to save his children) and wasn't able to release the pain. Whenever he was reminded that his boys were gone, he'd immediately go into self-blame, guilt, and shame and ruthlessly beat himself up for the horrible tragedy he had caused. But when he finally expressed his emotions stemming from the events of that day, he realized that he had not done anything "wrong" and in fact had done everything humanly possible to save his sons. This reframing was only possible because he had completed the Fritz. Before reframing the loss, he could actively avoid the sadness. Reframing required him to accept that his boys were gone. This acceptance was the most difficult part of the Fritz, as it usually is for people with trauma or grief. Just as when he was asked to purposely remember and when asked to say goodbye, he missed the appointment. Eventually though, with some encouragement, he confronted the sadness, felt it fully, and released it. Avoidance really is the archenemy of healing, and I hope that Jim's story communicates how it can have a negative impact on your own healing.

Questions for Comprehension

—

What are the three best ideas that you gleaned from this chapter?

_____

_____

_____

_____

_____

What type of action do you believe is necessary to help actualize these ideas?

_____

_____

_____

_____

_____

How did you execute your plan?

_____

_____

_____

_____

_____

What is the result of your efforts?

_____

_____

_____

_____

_____

Chapter Eleven

Finishing Your
Unfinished Business

•

"Yesterday... All my troubles seemed so far away.
Now it looks as though they're here to stay."
—The Beatles

"THE SIX-PACK" AND WHAT TO DO WITH OTHER UNFINISHED BUSINESS

While the majority of this book has focused on trauma (most of which would qualify as PTSD) or grief, the process that these severely traumatized individuals used is applicable for people who are dealing with a wide range of less catastrophic situations. Trauma is trauma; and it doesn't matter whether you want to heal from a parent who abandoned you or friends you've lost, you can use the Fritz to achieve your goals. I'd like to share the story of Jeff, who in order to make peace with the final days of his life, needed to address unfinished business from his past.

Jeff was seventy-one, and his traumatic event was the Vietnam War. It was so many years ago that Jeff was certain he was finally free of its chokehold on his happiness. Well, sort of. But he had lost three friends in six months, two of whom had been in-country when he was. Jeff wanted to cry for each one of these friends, but feared that if he did, he might never stop. He knew the reservoir of emotional tears flows like a mighty river, and he could only hope that the dam would hold up for the rest of his days.

Jeff didn't attend the funerals of these friends for fear of being overly emotional. He meant no disrespect to their wives and families—in fact, he sent enormous floral arrangements in lieu of his appearing personally. He just couldn't trust himself to maintain his composure.

Jeff and his wife, Carol, were having some communication issues—nothing too bad, really. She had benefited so much from therapy over the years that she insisted that he join her for a little lightweight couples' counseling to improve their relationship. After fifty years of avoiding "damn shrinks," he heard me speak at a local fundraiser and thought, "Why not give it a try, at least we'll have some laughs."

And laugh we did about the insanity of Vietnam, politics, the aging process, etc., until Jeff found out that he really wanted to cry about so many things. In fact, it didn't take him long to realize that there were sensitive areas in his life that aroused a very sad sentiment and embarrassed the former Marine by repeatedly reducing him to sobbing. Any one of these topics could render Jeff speechless, tears flowing, stammering about how he hated "being a seventy-one-year-old crybaby."

There were at least six issues in his life that we quickly dubbed, "the six-pack" that he had never finished, all of which had the power to instigate sobbing. Curiously, none of them were combat-related. In fact, none of the six were what we might label a "trauma," but each event (or Jeff's perception thereof) brought him into a place of deep sadness and brokenness. The totality of this six-pack had the capacity to bring forth tears, with the Kleenex box in one hand, several tissues in the other, evidence of the unfinished pain in his life.

One of the six-pack of unfinished issues involved a good friend of his named Gary, a guy with whom he had grown up. He had many a drinking story with Gary before Jeff finally stopped drinking in '97. But Jeff had quit talking to Gary ten years ago because he had caught Gary in a lie. And if there was one thing Jeff couldn't handle, it was a lie. Interestingly, the lie didn't impact Jeff at all. It was a lie about the way Gary had lost his job. He was embarrassed, it seemed, and didn't want anyone to know the truth. So, for that reason, he fudged the explanation of why he had been terminated and tried to sell it to Jeff. Jeff had found out the truth shortly thereafter and hadn't uttered a word to him since. But now, with the mere mention of Gary's name, Jeff was emptying my Kleenex box again.

After Vietnam, Jeff had come home and tried his hand at relationships. Each and every effort ended in disaster, and Jeff knew he was to blame each time. The drinking, the explosive rage, the anxiety, the jealousy—he was impossible to live with as a young hothead. Most of those relationships ultimately meant nothing to him until this one young lady, Nancy, who was pregnant with Jeff's child—something that had inspired true joy in Jeff's case—had planned on living life with Jeff and their baby. But Jeff couldn't commit to Nancy that he would marry her or have a monogamous relationship with her. He was afraid to keep his part of the bargain. So one day, Jeff's girlfriend decided to abort the child—she figured if he wouldn't commit, she didn't want to be saddled with the responsibility of raising a child on her own.

Jeff found out that his "child" had been aborted and felt devastated to lose what would have been his first child. Later, to add to his sense of despair, his new girlfriend, Carol, who soon after became his wife, found out that she was biologically incapable of childbirth. In other words, Jeff would not be having children, and he had missed his only chance to sire a child.

And there were other unresolved issues. Jeff's father wasn't to blame for most of his life's issues and disappointments. But secretly Jeff blamed his father for everything because his dad had left the family when Jeff was fifteen. His parents had always been fighting, but in Jeff's mind, Dad had left, and mom had stayed—it was clear who was the bad guy. Jeff hated his dad his entire adult life and would not return any of the old man's letters or phone calls. Then one day, Jeff's sister relayed that their dad had died at sixty-nine years old of a coronary event. "F*** him," Jeff thought, but that's not how it felt. He realized that he had blown his chance to reconcile with his only father. And now it was too late, he'd go to his grave feeling ashamed of having been too damn proud to reach out to his father and connect with the old man. Or would he?

Jeff quickly recognized that marital bickering was just a symptom of the real issue. He had a six-pack of unfinished issues in his life, all of which broke his fragile heart and cumulatively left him on the brink of an emotional meltdown whenever he broached any of them—three deceased friends, none of whom he had ever told how much he loved them, one estranged friend who had lied to Jeff for self-protection, one aborted child, and one deceased father who had longed to connect with his son for thirty years.

Once we had an identity—the six-pack—for his unfinished pains in the past, I challenged him to come to therapy by himself, without his wife Carol. We had a simple goal: Finish the six-pack. He laughed, of course, because in his drinking days that might have only taken half an hour, but now, he claimed, I might as well play the theme song for "Mission Impossible." How could he ever feel better if five of the six people in question were dead? "Shouldn't I be scheduling sessions with the Long Island Medium instead of you?" he quipped.

I opted to begin with the low hanging fruit: calling his friend whom he hadn't spoken to and tell him in his own words how much he missed him;

explain how sensitive he was to people lying after feeling like his father had lied to him by leaving and like his country had lied to him by sending him to a war he couldn't win, and tell his friend he was sorry and forgave him. And plan to go see his friend, and for God's sake, reconcile that relationship with Gary. Predictably, it only took one phone call to right that ship, and plans were made for the old buddies to get together at the next high school reunion that coming September.

The three amigos—his recent friends who had passed in the last six months—were next. I offered Jeff the options of, you guessed it, writing letters or imagery, and Jeff had a great idea of his own. Not one to waste resources in battle, money, or board games, he figured he'd do an imagery process where he could see all three guys at once. "You know, say goodbye to them, bust their balls, joke, we will all laugh and cry together. That way I won't feel so damned foolish using all of your tissues." As advertised, Jeff cried me a river that session, but he could hear the guys all joking about the next life. "We are not afraid of Hell," one said, "because we've already been to Vietnam." "I'm not afraid either," said the guy who didn't go; "After all, I've been divorced three times." There was alternating laughter and tears throughout the imagery, culminating finally in the men getting together to shake each other's hands in a type of impromptu circle. "But then a funny thing happened," said Jeff; "We traded in our handshakes for a giant group hug, something we'd never do in real life. But you know what, none of us wanted to let go. It was like that Billy Joel song... And we will all go down together."[57]

Jeff knew that he wanted to write a letter to the mother of his aborted child and apologize for his contributions toward destroying the only opportunity he'd ever had to be a father. In the letter, he told her that he'd realized that less than consciously, he was hoping she would go through with the abortion because he believed that his father had failed in that role, and Jeff knew he probably wouldn't do any better than his old man had. Now admittedly, saying this to the child that never was born was the single hardest thing he'd ever done in his life. "How do you apologize when you are guilty of removing someone's entire life just because you are too chicken to make mistakes?" But that's just what Jeff did, all in letter form. In fact, he ended his letter (to the unborn child he believed would have been his son) in the following manner: "Junior, I can't even ask you to forgive me for my cowardly behavior. Instead, I'd like to ask you for a second chance—will you save me a spot in heaven, son, where maybe I can play catch with you or take you fishing? I'll bet they've got some pretty cool go-karts in heaven. What do you say son, can we go for a ride together sometime?" At this point, the psychologist also needed a tissue, as he felt a little something welling up in his eyes also. It seemed to be a combination of incredible sadness and heartfelt joy, as Jeff was finally giving himself permission to be "okay" with the abortion and the loss of the child who never was.

But perhaps the biggest challenge for Jeff was to finally meet and confront his long-estranged father. We saved him for last. Jeff knew that he wanted to see his father in person, so imagery, again, was the treatment of choice. After an initial relaxation induction, Jeff met his father at the Little League field where Jeff used to play; his dad came to every one of his games, even if it meant leaving work early. Jeff had thought he might begin by telling his old man off, or worse, hearing his dad yell at him, "Why the hell didn't you call me!"

But he imagined none of that. The two men rushed to each other, and each threw their arms around the other one, holding tightly while crying and whispering, "I'm sorry, I love you, I love you too," for almost twelve straight minutes. There was no blaming, accusing, excusing, or justifying, just two fully grown yet tearful men releasing their hurt, sadness, and fear, and forgiving one another for running away from each other "like scared little sissies," Jeff said. But both men found the courage to reach out to each other—at least in imagery—and release all the toxicity that Jeff had carried for 56 years of silence. He was finally free to release his dad. Forgive his dad. Love his dad. Finally, it was okay.

Two months later, Jeff died at the age of seventy-two from a heart attack—just like his dad. But while Jeff experienced cardiac failure, he now possessed a pure heart, one that was free of hatred, guilt, and self-contempt. Jeff was finally free!

Perhaps there are unfinished chapters in your life. I can only hope that you now possess the understanding and the tools to take on the challenge of finishing your pain in the past.

Questions for Comprehension

—

What are the three best ideas that you gleaned from this chapter?

_____

_____

_____

_____

_____

What type of action do you believe is necessary to help actualize these ideas?

_____

_____

_____

_____

_____

How did you execute your plan?

_____

_____

_____

_____

_____

What is the result of your efforts?

_____

_____

_____

_____

_____

Chapter Twelve

Out of the Traumatic Past and Into a Better Future

"I will survive."
—Gloria Gaynor

OUT OF THE PAST AND INTO A BETTER FUTURE

◇

As sad as some of the stories I've related are, I see this book as one of great joy, promise, and healing. The stories are indeed gruesome at times, featuring as they do the death of children, combat horrors, sexual abuse, betrayal, abandonment, and unrequited love. Yet the only reason the stories are worth telling is this: despite their awful experiences, the people were able to recover. The common denominator of each story? Someone endured a horrible incident, and yet, by applying the healing principles of the Fritz, each person could release the trauma and make peace with his or her past.

Instead of being trapped in grappling with issues like smoldering guilt, lingering addictions, and suffocating anxiety, these individuals are now free from the ravages of their unresolved trauma. They are no longer haunted by their traumas, having put away the ugliness forever.

Recently, while jogging on the beach, I stopped long enough to talk to a former client who had presenting issues of childhood abuse and multiple personalities. I had not seen her for at least five years, and felt compelled to ask, "How are you doing with your childhood?"

She looked puzzled, ripped off her Oakley designer sunglasses, and stated, "You know we put that away years ago. It's long over with, Dr. Cortman. You know that!"

Of course, that was what I wanted to hear, but a part of me needed the reassurance that when the past is put away, it's resolved for good. It doesn't have to be renewed every five years like a driver's license. The splinter is out, and the middle toe is forever better.

But maybe your pain in the past was not as traumatic or dramatic as a fatal car accident or a devil worshiping cult. And yet you were every bit as tormented by your unfinished past. Trauma is personal; what might only be a minor problem for one person is a major issue for another.

Dawn presented with symptoms of depression that robbed her of the joy and confidence that her work and motherhood would have otherwise afforded her. The problem was a toxic, self-deprecating mindset, largely the byproduct of perceived inferiority during childhood. After Dawn's older sister died in a traumatic accident when Dawn was young, her mother had said, "I wish it had been you that died and Donna was still here."

Dawn needed to purge the statement—and the concomitant shame. After sharing the story of a childhood of "not measuring up," Dawn elected to write a letter to her deceased mother to express and release what it felt like to be an eleven-year-old daughter whose mother wished she were dead instead of her sister. Dawn was also able to understand that her mother's statement was made under the influence of grief, rage, and alcohol, a poisonous threesome by any measure. By telling her mother how it felt (in a letter) and understanding that her mother had been speaking from the Bermuda Triangle of devastating emotions and liquor, Dawn could release that shame forever and finally heal from her depression. She remains at peace with her mother, her sister. and her childhood belief that she'd never measure up. And Dawn is no longer "a depressed client."

Her story is painful, to be sure, but it lacks the horror, say, of John's account of the Vietnamese child. The Fritz will work to heal whatever you may be carrying from the past, great or small, as long as you feel, express, and choose to release your pain. And that means accepting it for whatever it is instead of trying to make the past different from what it was.

All my years of practice tell me that the Fritz will work for you, whether your dreams were thwarted by a controlling parent or adult; you were cheated by a former business partner; your career was snuffed out by ALS, CMT, or MS; or the love of your life believed you weren't the love of his. There is no shortage of hurt, disappointment, or loss in an eighty-year life span, including thousands of people and possessions that you will need to say goodbye to and release.

In a class I once attended on aging, the professor stated the following with authority: The people who fare the best in their older years are those who understand the losses they must endure, as well as the need to replace those losses. In other words, when your dog Duke dies, it's time to conduct a ceremony, grieve your loss, and tearfully bury him in the backyard. Three months later—say hello to "Sparky," your new Shih Tzu puppy. Likewise, if your wife leaves you for your best friend, you must again feel your pain, sadness, and anger, say goodbye to your losses. and eventually replace your wife (and your best friend). It is the great circle of life, or more accurately, the great circle of love.

Let this be your mantra: love, lose, grieve, love again, lose again, grieve again.

And whenever there is loss or trauma, the principles of the Fritz will prove to be effective. Remember the Fritz can be implemented in as many ways as you can imagine, as long as the bottom line is letting go and saying goodbye.

Based on my practice, the two best ways to implement the five steps of the Fritz are letter-writing and guided imagery. Anyone can write a farewell letter anytime, but ideally, your letter should feature four elements:

- What happened

- How it felt at the time

- How it affected you since

- What you are going to do to let it go

Letter writing works, provided you are prepared to say goodbye.

Guided imagery, a technique I find unparalleled in its effectiveness, will afford you the opportunity to envision whatever you need to experience for a very realistic immersion into pain, release, and then closure. This is an extraordinarily effective manner by which to say goodbye to a trauma that has continued to hold you in its clutches, be it a car accident, a combat scene, or a sexual assault. This technique is effective in allowing you to say goodbye to a "lost" person who lingers painfully in your mind because some aspect of their life is unfinished with respect to you. While you can effectively imagine anything you like in the privacy of your own imagination, using the services of an experienced mental health professional is often a good idea. A professional experienced in employing this technique can help you create the necessary scenario with great effectiveness. If you can't make guided imagery work on your own, contact a professional to help you visualize the experience and then release its hold on your life.

There are of course other ways to achieve this objective. Some of you may employ the Fritz by going to the graveyard and sitting near your grandfather's grave in order to recall, feel, and express your feelings to him.

You say goodbye to him or whatever painful issue is associated with him in an effort to put grandpa in a healthy place in your mind and in your life.

I've suggested the option of calling on a professional to help you with guided imagery, but you shouldn't shy away from using this technique because you're bound and determined to put the suggestions in this book into practice on your own. It's often the combination of the work you do by yourself and the guidance a professional provides that helps you heal. If in employing the five steps of the Fritz you cannot find the peace that comes from releasing something painful or traumatic, consider employing the services of a mental health professional. If you have complex PTSD or chronic, unrelenting PTSD (or any type of mental illness), you are more likely to require professional treatment.

On your own or with a professional, this key goal remains constant: make peace with the trauma, finish the unfinished business, and come to acceptance regarding the pain in the past. Of course, saying goodbye does not require a one-time release. You may gradually release people you love over time. This is normal. *But the Fritz is indicated for people who are stuck in trauma or grieving.* I emphasize this point because it's crucial to know if you're stuck, and when you're stuck, to reach for the Fritz.

I give you this remarkable technique to help you as an individual but also in the hope that it will change the landscape of treatment for unresolved trauma, loss, unfinished business, and PTSD. Those who suffer from unrelenting PTSD or a life of unhappiness due to an unfinished aspect of childhood truly deserve the opportunity to achieve peace. If this book can help you realize this goal, I will have succeeded.

References

1. Stewart, A. (1976). Time Passages. On *Year of the Cat* [CD]. Los Angeles, CA: Davlen Studios.

2. Jeffreys, M. (2017). *Clinician's Guide to Medication for PTSD*. U.S. Department of Veterans Affairs, Washington, DC. https://www.ptsd.va.gov/professional/treatment/overview/clinicians-guide-to-medications-for-ptsd.asp

3. National Center for PTSD. (2018). *Understand PTSD and PTSD Treatment. https://www.ptsd.va.gov/public/understanding_ptsd/booklet.pdf*

4. James Framo. (1982). Lecture on Psychological treatment on Trauma. United States International University, San Diego, CA.

5. Selye H. (1978). *The Stress of Life*. New York, NY: McGraw-Hill.

6. Szabo, S., Tache, Y., Somogyi, A. (2012). The legacy of Hans Selye and the origins of stress research: a retrospective 75 years after his landmark brief letter to the editor of Nature. *Stress, 15*, 472–478. DOI: 10.3109/10253890.2012.710919.

7. Bremner, J. D. (2006). Traumatic stress: effects on the brain. *Dialogues in Clinical Neuroscience, 8*(4), 445–461.

8. Vermetten, E., Bremner, J. D. (2002). Circuits and systems in stress. II. Applications to neurobiology and treatment in posttraumatic stress disorder. *Depress Anxiety, 16*(1), 14–38.

9. Pitman, R. K., Shin, L. M., Rauch, S. L. (2001) Investigating the pathogenesis of posttraumatic stress disorder with neuroimaging. *Journal of Clinical Psychiatry, 62*, 47–54.

10. Elzinga, B. M., Schmahl, C. S., Vermetten, E., et al. (2003). Increased cortisol responses to the stress of traumatic reminders in abuse-related PTSD. *Neuropsychopharmacology, 28,* 1656–1665.

11. Gola, H., Engler, H., Schauer, M., Adenauer, H., Riether, C., Kolassa, S., ...Kolassa, I.T. (2012). Victims of rape show increased cortisol responses to trauma reminders: a study in individuals with war- and torture-related PTSD. *Psychoneuroendocrinilogy, 37*(2), 213–220.

12. Koenigs, M., & Grafman, J. (2009). Post-traumatic stress disorder: The role of medial prefrontal cortex and amygdala. *The Neuroscientist : A Review Journal Bringing Neurobiology, Neurology and Psychiatry, 15*(5), 540–548. http://doi.org/10.1177/1073858409333072

13. Beck, Judith. (2011). *CBT and Beck: Cognitive Behavior Therapy: Basics and Beyond. 2nd edition.* New York, NY: The Guildford Press.

14. Akhtar, M. (2008). *What is Self-Efficacy? Bandura's 4 Sources of Efficacy Beliefs.* Retrieved from http://positivepsychology.org.uk/self-efficacy-definition-bandura-meaning/

15. Ucros, C. (2008). Mood state-dependent memory: A meta-analysis. *Cognition and Emotion, 3*(2), 139–169.

16. Deveral, J. (2016). *Why do survivors of disasters feel guilt about surviving?* Retrieved from http://survivor-story.com/why-survivors-of-tragedies-feel-guilt

17. Kar, N. (2011). Cognitive behavioral therapy for the treatment of post-traumatic stress disorder: a review. *Neuropsychiatric Disease and Treatment, 7,* 167–181. http://doi.org/10.2147/NDT.S10389

18. Schottenbauer, M.A., Glass, C.R., Arnkoff, D.B., Tendick, V., Gray, S.,H. (2008). Nonresponse and dropout rates in outcome studies on PTSD: Review and methodological considerations. *Psychiatry, 71*(2), 134–168.

19. Freud, A. (1937). *The Ego and the Mechanisms of Defence*. London: Pub. by L. and Virginia Woolf at the Hogarth Press, and the Institute of Psychoanalysis.

20. Jordan, Karin. (2008). *The Quick Theory Reference Guide: A Resource for Expert and Novice Mental Health Professionals*. New York, NY: Nova Science Publishers, Inc.

21. Seligman, L., Reichenberg, L. (2010) *Theories of Counseling and Psychotherapy: Systems, Strategies, and Skills*. Boston, MA: Prentice Hall.

22. Kushner, H. S. (1981). *When Bad Things Happen to Good People*. New York, NY: Schocken Books.

23. Sayed, D. (2014). *Forgiveness in Different Religious Traditions*. Retrieved from http://blogs.shu.edu/diplomacyresearch/2014/05/06/forgiveness-in-different-religious-traditions/

24. Twain, M. Web reference. Retrieved from https://www.goodreads.com/quotes/109049-anger-is-an-acid-that-can-do-more-harm-to

25. Weir, K. (2017). *Forgiveness can improve mental and physical health*. Retrieved from http://www.apa.org/monitor/2017/01/ce-corner.aspx

26. Simon, S., Simon, S. (1990). *Forgiveness: How to Make Peace With Your Past and Get On With Your Life*. New York, NY: Grand Central Publishing.

27. Livgren, K. (1977). Dust in the Wind. On *Point of Know Return* [CD]. Nashville, TN: Kirshner.

28. Najavits, L. M., Weiss, R. D. and Shaw, S. R. (1997). The Link Between Substance Abuse and Posttraumatic Stress Disorder in Women. *The American Journal on Addictions, 6*: 273–283. DOI:10.1111/j.1521-0391.1997.tb00408.x

29. Triffleman, E. G., Marmar, C. R., Delucchi, K. L., & Ronfeldt, H. (1995). Childhood trauma and posttraumatic stress disorder in substance abuse inpatients. *Journal of Nervous and Mental Disease, 183*(3), 172–176. http://dx.doi.org/10.1097/00005053-199503000-00008

30. Deykin, E. Y., Buka, S. L. (1997). Prevalence and risks factors for posttraumatic stress disorder among chemically dependent adolescents. *The American Journal of Psychiatry. 154*(6), 752–757.

31. Felitti, V. J. (2003). The Origins of Addiction: Evidence from the Adverse Childhood Experiences Study. English version of the article published in Germany as: Felitti VJ. Ursprünge des Suchtverhaltens— *Evidenzen aus einer Studie zu belastenden Kindheitserfahrungen. Praxis der Kinderpsychologie und Kinderpsychiatrie, 52,* 547–559.

32. Becker, A. (2013). The single greatest preventable cause of mental illness. Quote from Dr. Steven Sharfstein. Retrieved from http://wellmore.org/news-info/news-releases/the-single-greatest-preventable-cause-of-mental-illness/

33. Perls, F. (1973). *The Gestalt Approach & Eye Witness to Therapy.* Oxford, England: Science & Behavior Books.

34. Kirschman, E. (2017). *Cops and PTSD.* Retrieved from https://www.psychologytoday.com/us/blog/cop-doc/201706/cops-and-ptsd-0

35. O' Sullivan, G. (1971). Alone Again. On *Himself* [CD]. London, England: MAM.

36. Terr, L. (1994). *Unchained Memories: True Stories of Traumatic Memories, Lost and Found.* New York, NY: Basic Books.

37. Henley, D. (1988). The Heart of the Matter. On *The End of the Innocence* [CD]. Santa Monica, CA: Geffen Records.

38. Henley, D. (1988). The End of Innocence. On *The End of Innocence* [CD]. Santa Monica, CA: Geffen Records.

39. W., Bill. (1976). *Alcoholics Anonymous: The Story of How Many Thousands of Men and Women Have Recovered from Alcoholism.* New York, NY: Alcoholics Anonymous World Services.

40. Hall, K. (2012). *Understanding Validation: A Way to Communicate Acceptance.* Retrieved from https://www.psychologytoday.com/us/blog/pieces-mind/201204/understanding-validation-way-communicate-acceptance

41. Ackerman, R. (2002). *Perfect Daughters (Revised Edition): Adult Daughters of Alcoholics.* Deerfield Beach, FL: Health Communications, Inc.

42. Post, P., Wrisberg, C., Mullins, S. (2010). A Field Test of the Influence of Pre-Game Imagery on Basketball Free Throw Shooting. *Journal of Imagery Research in Sport and Physical Activity*, 5(1).

43. Wolfson, R. (1993). *The Phases of Jewish Bereavement.* Retrieved from https://www.myjewishlearning.com/article/the-phases-of-jewish-bereavement/

44. Joel, B. (1981). Say Goodbye to Hollywood. On *Songs in the Attic* [CD]. Milwaukee, WI: Columbia Records.

45. Barnes, D., Carlisi, J., Steele, L., Van Zant, D. (1984). If I'd Been The One. On *Tour de Force* [CD]. Doraville, GA: A&M Records.

46. Cortman, C., Shinitzky, H. (2010). *Your Mind: An Owner's Manual For A Better Life.* Franklin Lakes, NJ: Career Press.

47. Seligman, M. E. P. (2006). *Learned Optimism: How to Change Your Mind and Your Life.* New York, NY: Vintage Books.

48. Kohlberg, L. (1981). *The Philosophy of Moral Development: Moral Stages and the Idea of Justice.* San Francisco, CA: Harper & Row.

49. Lazare, A. (2004). *On Apology.* New York, NY: Oxford University Press.

50. McCartney, P. (1969). Yesterday. On *Abbey Road* [CD]. London, England: Apple Records.

51. National Center for PTSD. (2016). *Complex PTSD*. Retrieved from https://www.ptsd.va.gov/professional/ptsd-overview/complex-ptsd.asp

52. Van der Kolk, B. A. (2014). *The Body Keeps the Score: Brain, Mind, and Body in the Healing of Trauma*. New York, NY: Viking.

53. Lampert, L. (2016). *Burnout, Compassion Fatigue, and Secondary Post Traumatic Stress*. Retrieved from https://www.ausmed.com/articles/burnout-fatigue-post-traumatic-stress/

54. Lawson, D. (2018). *Understanding and treating survivors of incest*. Counseling Today, Knowledge Sharing. Retrieved from https://ct.counseling.org/2018/03/understanding-treating-survivors-incest/

55. M. Bergman, A. Bergman, M. Hamlisch. (1974). The Way We Were. On *The Way We Were*. [CD] New York, NY: Columbia.

56. McCartney, P., Lennon, J. (1965). Yesterday. On *Help!* [CD]. London, England: EMI Studios.

57. Joel, B. (1982). Goodbye Saigon. On *The Nylon Curtain*. [CD] New York, NY: Columbia.

58. Gaynor, G. (1978). I Will Survive. On *Love Tracks* [CD]. London, England: Polydor Records.

Appendix One

The Fritz and How It Compares to Other Trauma-Focused Therapies

By Joseph Walden

Eye movement desensitization and reprocessing (EMDR) and Prolonged Exposure (PE) are the two main competitors of the Fritz. I'll do my best to describe these alternatives and compare them to what I am recommending.

Eye Movement Desensitization and Reprocessing (EMDR)

EMDR was developed by American psychologist Francine Shapiro in the late 1980s for the treatment of post-traumatic stress disorder (PTSD).[1] The therapist uses an external stimulus to reduce the affective distress associated with the traumatic experience. The most common is bilateral eye-movements, but hand-tapping or audio stimulation are also used. Clients will be trained how to engage in bilateral eye-movements and then will be asked to engage in this behavior while they are telling their story of trauma. Several research studies have found that EMDR is an effective treatment, and the American Psychiatric Association[2] has designated EMDR as an effective treatment for PTSD. Treatment is broken down into eight phases. The first phase is a history-taking session, essentially an intake session to identify problem areas and past traumas. Phase two ensures that the client has adequate and healthy coping skills before old traumatic injuries are stirred up. Phases three through six are related to vivid imagery of the traumatic memory, identifying negative beliefs about the self, and processing uncovered emotions. Phase seven is closure and monitoring the

ent experiences throughout the coming week. Phase eight is
urrent issues that elicit distress. For more information on this
please refer to Shapiro's book, *Eye Movement Desensitization*
cessing (EMDR) Therapy: Basic Principles, Protocols, and
Procedures.[3]

While research studies have concluded that EMDR is effective in clinical
trials, the mechanism of this success was until recently mostly unknown.
Lilienfeld and Arkowitz (2012) state that completing EMDR is better than
doing nothing, but not as effective as other trauma-focused therapies, in
this case things like prolonged exposure. They went on to say that the
results that proved effective likely were due to the exposure, rather than
the "eye movement."[4]

My personal conclusions regarding EMDR stem from my clients who have
completed this protocol. While talking to a therapist, learning various
coping skills, and feeling "somewhat" better are positive, the traumas tend
to creep back into the mind.

There are a number of significant differences between EMDR and the Fritz.
Obviously, there has been no discussion of "eye movement" in this entire
book up until this point. There is a reason for that: eye movement isn't a
requirement for healing, just as keeping your eyes fixed on a single point
isn't a requirement for healing. Missing from EMDR are the releasing and
reframing steps of the Fritz. These two steps help people achieve the very
important feeling of closure. With closure, the trauma or grief is over. That
chapter of life is closed.

There are some elements of EMDR that are present in the steps of the
Fritz. For example, EMDR typically includes guided imagery back into the
period that the trauma was experienced, as does the Fritz. However, the
mere element of exposure is inadequate to fully treat trauma. And while
the clients I've worked with who experienced EMDR before seeing me were

exposed to their traumas, they repeatedly told me that they still felt as they had an open wound. Obviously, this is not the goal of the Fritz, and while EMDR is better than no treatment, I don't believe it to be nearly as effective to treat trauma.

Prolonged Exposure (PE)

Prolonged Exposure (PE) was originally developed by Dr. Edna Foa, who has been the director of the Center for the Treatment and Study of Anxiety since the late 1990s. Prolonged exposure is commonly used to help people confront various fears and phobias. Most people want to avoid things that remind them of trauma (Mr. Avoidance). Since avoidance is thought to maintain the fear, exposure, obviously, is the opposite.

Prolonged exposure is a manualized treatment that occurs over the course of a three-month period. Usually, there are nine to twelve sessions, lasting about ninety minutes each.[5] There are two types of exposure, imaginal and in vivo. Imaginal exposure is exposure in one's imagination. The client imagines the traumatic event and is thereby exposed to a somewhat less threatening version of the trauma, simply because imagination is not reality. The client and therapist discuss any emotions that arise. In vivo exposure is confronting the feared stimuli outside of therapy, in the real world. As an example, someone with PTSD from a motor vehicle accident might be required to go sit in their car, drive locally, and eventually make an extended trip. The goal here is to get the client to challenge him/herself in a graduated fashion to remove associated fears.

Prolonged Exposure (PE) is largely regarded at the "gold standard" of trauma treatments. It had been shown to be effective in treating combat veterans, sexual assault survivors, refugees, and adult survivors of childhood abuse in all kinds of ethnic and racial groups.[6] While prolonged exposure is a good treatment, there is something that is often overlooked. Dropout rates for those attending prolonged exposure therapy vary greatly, but some studies suggest rates as high as 50 percent.[7] Several studies have looked at trauma treatments for PTSD, and again, the dropout rate of 20 percent is concerning.[8]

Prolonged exposure can indeed treat PTSD, and research tends to support that. Some of the elements of PE are similar to the Fritz, primarily the exposure element. Clients going through the Fritz will have to expose themselves to their traumatic memories in the "remember" and "express" steps of the Fritz. However, in my humble opinion, merely exposing yourself to these trauma memories over and over again is unnecessary punishment. This unnecessary punishment, I think, accounts for the high dropout rate of PE. As compared to the Fritz, during which the "exposure" element only occurs once and then the process of release begins; no unnecessary prolonged and continued exposures are needed.

Final thoughts on EMDR and PE

While both EMDR and PE have some supporting research, they both have limitations. I believe that the Fritz addresses these limitations. As stated earlier, as you've gone through this book, I've never once mentioned your eye movement. It simply isn't necessary, because eye movement has little to do with healing from trauma. While the exposure element of PE is required for healing (and included in the Fritz), more is needed for closure and acceptance to occur. Reframing the trauma and releasing the trauma help people finish the unfinished business in their life. Adding these steps is what separates this treatment from others, and it is what helps people gain closure and move on with their lives.

References: Appendix One

1. EMDR Institute, Inc. (2018). What is EMDR? Retrieved fromhttp:// www.emdr.com/what-is-emdr/

2. EMDR International Association. (2018). Does EMDR really work? Retrieved from https://emdria.site-ym.com/?122

3. Shapiro, F. (2001). *Eye Movement Desensitization and Reprocessing (EMDR) Therapy: Basic Principles, Protocols, and Procedures. Second Edition*. New York, NY: Guilford Press.

4. Lilienfeld, S., Arkowitz, H. (2012). *EMDR: Taking a closer look. Can moving your eyes back and forth help to ease anxiety?* Retrieved from https://www.scientificamerican.com/article/emdr-taking-a-closer-look/

5. Foa, E. B., Hembree, E. A., & Rothbaum, B. O. (2007). *Prolonged Exposure Therapy for PTSD: Emotional Processing of Traumatic Experiences, Therapist Guide*. New York, NY: Oxford University Press.

6. Eftekhari, A., Stines, L. R., & Zoellner, L. A. (2006). Do You Need To Talk About It? Prolonged Exposure for the Treatment of Chronic PTSD. *The Behavior Analyst Today, 7*(1), 70–83.

7. Cottraux J, Note I, Yao SN, de Mey Guillard C, Bonasse FCO, Djamoussian D, Mollard E, et al. (2008). *Randomized controlled comparison of cognitive behavior therapy with Rogerian supportive therapy in chronic posttraumatic stress disorder: A 2-year follow-up. Psychotherapy and Psychosomatics, 77*(2):101–110.

8. Imel, Z. E., Laska, K., Jakcupcak, M., & Simpson, T. L. (2013). Meta-analysis of Dropout in Treatments for Posttraumatic Stress Disorder. *Journal of Consulting and Clinical Psychology, 81*(3), 394–404. http://doi.org/10.1037/a0031474

Appendix Two

Our Top Ten Coping Skills

By Joseph Walden

Completing the Fritz is helpful, but there still might be other things that you need help with. Here is a list of my top ten coping skills. By no mean is this list comprehensive, and it isn't intended to be, but if I had to pick only ten, it would be these ten.

1. Alcoholics Anonymous, Narcotics Anonymous, and Other Twelve-Step Programs

The twelve steps of Alcoholics Anonymous (AA) are the foundation of countless stories of sobriety. These time-tested pearls of wisdom have stood unchanged since Bill Wilson and Dr. Bob Smith co-authored them in 1935.[1] Many therapists don't appreciate AA, NA, and other twelve-step programs, but they can be extremely helpful, whether alone or in conjunction with psychotherapy. The results are hard to discount: AA has helped millions of alcoholics start and maintain recovery. For those who are reading this book and who have struggled with your own addiction, please read the next few paragraphs. For those in a relationship with someone with an addiction, I will detail other groups that may be helpful.

There are so many benefits to AA, but I'll keep the list relatively short. First, AA is everywhere. You can search Google for "AA meetings in _____ county" and find meetings in nearly every county throughout the United States, or even internationally. In larger cities, there are AA meetings literally every hour. In rural areas, AA meetings are frequently held at local churches. Ease of accessibility is perhaps the greatest benefit of AA. As a psychologist, I work diligently to make myself available to my clients, but I cannot be available every day of the week, let alone every hour (as AA meetings are in some places), like an AA meeting can.

Another benefit of AA is that is totally free: no insurance, no copays, nor any in-network or out-of-network benefits to worry about. For many people struggling with addiction, stable employment and insurance simply aren't available. Without insurance and a stable income, access to counseling may not be a possibility. But thankfully, community resources such as AA exist that can help with recovery from alcohol or drugs.

Accessibility and free availability are great, but the content, sponsorship, twelve steps, and sense of community are equally helpful. Knowing that you are not alone in the recovery process is so important. Meeting others who are working on recovery provides a valuable resource to everyone who is in the group. "Old timers" in AA who have twenty or thirty years of sobriety help those who have been sober for two days. The ability to find a sponsor is an amazing addition to AA. Rehab centers work with clients to create a "sobriety" network, friends and family who will help with the client's recovery by not drinking around them. Having a sponsor in AA provides the person newly in recovery with someone who has "been there and done that." The twelve steps of AA are therapeutic in nature and can help people heal their own lives and those of the people around them. Earlier in the book, I explained how AA's "fearless moral inventory" is analogous to the four steps of forgiveness I recommend.

So why is AA included in the list of coping skills? For many people struggling with addiction, trauma is an underlying cause. AA is great, but it doesn't adequately address trauma (and it's not designed to do so). While removing chemically dependency is helpful, unless trauma is addressed, the likelihood of relapse is high. When pulling weeds from your garden, you have to get the roots. The trauma is the root, and the weed is addiction. If you have tried

AA or NA before with limited success but have now completed the Fritz, give AA a shot again. With the underlying root removed, the likelihood of remaining sober increases.

There are also other groups for people affected by addiction. Like AA, these groups are easily found on the internet. Al-Anon is designated for people who love someone who has an addiction, including spouses, husbands, wives, parents, girlfriends, and boyfriends. Loved ones find support, education about addiction, and information on how to set proper boundaries and how to love from a distance, if needed. ACoA stands for Adult Children of Alcoholics. Here, adult children find support, discuss how to cope, set boundaries, and practice their own recovery.

In addition to groups addressing substance addiction, there are other groups that might be beneficial. Similar in design to AA, Overeaters Anonymous (OA), Sexaholics Anonymous (SA), and Gamblers Anonymous (GA) all address potentially unhealthy coping strategies.

All in all, I'm a huge fan of twelve-step programs. With the underlying trauma or grief addressed and hopefully resolved using the Fritz, your chances of success in these groups increases drastically. So even if you have tried these groups before, give it a shot again. They have helped millions.

2. The Serenity Prayer

"God grant me the serenity to accept the things I cannot change, the courage to change the things I can, and the wisdom to know the difference."

There is so much wisdom in this single sentence that I've included it in this list. This expression is common in twelve-step programs and is often said before closing out each meeting. But it has other uses, too.

I often use the Serenity Prayer to explain healthy boundaries in interpersonal relationships. Let's start with the first part. As humans, we have almost scary limits on the amount of control we have and only limited things we can change. We have control over what we do with our hands, our feet, and what we say or don't say. But other than that, control is limited. You can do everything right and bad things can still happen. Being the best driver in the world won't stop someone from hitting your car. Be the perfect parent, and your child may still develop an addiction. Manage your diet, exercise regularly, never smoke or drink, and you may still develop cancer. You have responsibility for yourself only, and even when you do everything right, things still go wrong. For all the things that *you cannot change*, you need the *serenity of acceptance*.

Think about the last time you were frustrated with your boss, partner, or adult child, all people that you cannot change. Frustration with others can be a sign that you wish to change something that cannot be changed. If you have a child with an addiction, you have likely felt this. You want the best for your child, but ultimately, their sobriety is their journey, not yours. Try to change something that you can't, and the first consequence is frustration. The second consequence is likely to be anger or guilt. Jim felt he should bring his sons back to life. Instead, Jim needed the serenity to accept the loss.

Let's talk more about the second part of the prayer, *the courage the change the things I can*. It's hard to change almost any behavior. Getting a toddler to stop sucking their thumb, or for an adult, remaining sober from alcohol or starting a new diet are all challenging. What do people need to face challenges? Courage. Going to your first AA or NA meeting is scary; going to a gym for the first time is scary; breaking up with an abusive partner is scary. Again, all require courage. This is probably the most helpful reframe for people who find it difficult to do these behaviors. People who go to AA meetings and admit they struggle with addiction are brave. Telling your therapist that you were raped requires courage. Opening up to your therapist and discussing the rape in detail requires even more courage. This is why I prefer the expression "rape survivor" to "rape victim." Surviving after abuse, or surviving after someone you love has died, requires strength and courage.

The last part of the prayer is *the wisdom to know the difference*. The difference between what you can and cannot change is vast, and knowing the difference requires wisdom. This is one of those life lessons in which experience can be a brutal teacher, where the lesson will be learned after the class is taught. To summarize, we are in control of ourselves, and that is about all we can control. When people try to change other people, it is often frustrating and fruitless, and our efforts are likely best used in managing ourselves first.

3. Diaphragmatic Breathing

Earlier in the book, I mentioned that stress activates the "alarm switch" in your brain, causing your body to react accordingly. One of the most unpleasant symptoms of a panic attack is the feeling that you can't breathe, because you are breathing so hard. This is called hyperventilation. People do sometimes hyperventilate to the point that they faint. You may also have noticed that anxiety is sometimes accompanied by short, shallow breaths. This decreases the available oxygen in your bloodstream, and guess what? Your brain likes oxygen. In fact, your brain likes oxygen so much that if there is too little oxygen, the brain freaks out and creates the feeling of anxiety to warn you that something is very wrong.

That vicious cycle can continue, potentially indefinitely. You feel anxious, your respiration changes, your body becomes deoxygenated and freaks out, and you feel more anxious, thus completing the circle. But here's the good news, there is a simple and extremely effective way to break this cycle, and it's called diaphragmatic breathing.

The diaphragm is a dome-shaped muscle located at the base of your lungs; while it works with your abdominal muscles, it is responsible for pulling your lungs down, which fills them with air. You can feel it working right now—take a deep breath. It is right beneath your ribs and on top of your stomach; it separates the two. If you take a deep breath, you'll also learn that the diaphragm is a muscle that you can voluntarily control, which is great and important for the following exercise. Taking manual control over your breathing allows you to shift from the anxious, short, shallow breaths to longer, deeper, calming breaths. Taking deeper breaths (filling your lungs with air) allows more air into your lungs. where oxygen can be extracted and sent into the bloodstream. Oxygenating your body has a calming effect and breaks the above described cycle. So how do you do it?

1. Get into a comfortable position.

   a. If you do this in a chair, sit upright and find a balance where your spine is as straight as possible. Your torso should support itself in an upright stance. The goal here is to get into a position where you don't have to strain yourself to stay upright.

   b. If you are lying down, lie on your back with your head supported and held in place by a pillow. Again, the goal here is to find a position that requires little muscle involvement other than the ones used for breathing.

2. Place one hand on your chest and one on your stomach. Take a moment to observe which hand is moving more. If you are anxious, it is likely that the hand on your chest is moving more while the one on your stomach might not be moving at all. If the hand on your chest is moving more, this is a signal that you are taking shallow breaths and only filling the top third of your lungs.

3. Take control of the breath. Breathe in slowly through your nose. Keep taking in air until the hand on your stomach begins to move. You'll likely notice that moving the hand on your stomach requires longer, deeper breaths. Different authorities recommend different

amounts of time for these longer breaths, anywhere from five to ten seconds. As long as you are moving the hand on your stomach, it probably doesn't matter. But I would recommend taking your time. Imagine there is a candle in front of your mouth; you want to breathe out enough to move the flame, but not so quickly that you blow it out.

4. Continue this style of breathing for some time. At first, aiming for just a couple of minutes will be adequate and helpful. As you get more comfortable with this type of breathing, you can extend the amount of time you breathe this way to five minutes, ten minutes, or fifteen minutes, etc.

If you just did this exercise, how do you feel? I would guess that you feel better now than you did a few minutes ago. This is a very simple but highly effective way to manage anxiety, and one of my favorite parts is you can do this in public and no one will know.

4. The Five Questions for Rational Thinking[2]

The five questions for rational thinking were derived by Dr. Maxie Maultsby during his work as a psychiatric resident at the University of Wisconsin. The purpose of the five questions is to help people identify sensible thinking and behavior that keeps our own best interests in mind. The goal for the individual is to commit the five rules (or questions) in mind to ensure that you are always acting in your own self-interest. First, I'll list what the five questions are and then go into more depth regarding each.

The Five Questions for Rational Thinking

1. Is my thinking based on objective facts?

2. Will my thinking help me protect myself from probable harm?

3. Will my thinking here help me achieve my short- and long-term goals?

4. Will my thinking here help me avoid conflict with others?

5. Will my thinking help me feel the way I want to feel?

Is my thinking based on objective facts?

This question refers to how people think about what they consider to be facts and what they consider to be truth. Facts refer to objective reality, which exists whether anyone knows about it, likes it, or accepts it. What people consider to be true, however, is simply what they believe. The distinction may appear small, but when you really think about it, most emotional reactions are based on what is believed to be true, not on objective fact. If you believe your spouse is having an affair, you might become angry, but without proof, the affair is only your belief, not objective reality. Imagine an event, any event, being recorded by a video camera. Facts are seen on the recording. Anything that the camera cannot record is merely your opinion.

Will my thinking protect me from probable harm?

Because you are alive and reading this, you have a choice to make: to live self-destructively or to live self-protectively. Thinking, "I've only had a few drinks and I'm okay to drive home" exemplifies self-destructive thinking. A self-protective line of thinking might be, "I've only had a few drinks, but I should still call a cab just in case." Different lines of thinking result in helpful or harmful behaviors. Exploring the consequences of your thinking will be helpful for emotional health.

Will my thinking help me obtain my short- and long-term goals?

Hope is one of the primary forces behind all behavior. People go to school and pursue a higher education with the *hope* of obtaining a good job. People meet, date, and marry a partner with the *hope* that they will have a long, happy marriage. People go to therapy with the *hope* they will feel better. Most if not all of the things you do today are in some way related to what you want to do tomorrow or in the future.

Of the five questions, this one is especially important in addressing short-term and long-term concerns. For example, telling your boss how horrible he is might feel better in the short term, but losing your job is not good in the long term. Drinking after a stressful day may be a good short-term solution, but if relied on frequently, can develop into alcohol addiction, which is obviously not good for your long-term health. I use this line of questioning frequently with my clients. For the young boy who wants to become a surgeon, I say, "Great, you need to go to school today, pay attention, do the homework, and study. Then tomorrow, do it all again. And then the day after that, do it all again." For the alcoholic in recovery, I recommend AA meetings. Going to an AA meeting decreases the chances that you will drink today and helps you reach the long-term goal of sobriety.

All behavior is purposeful, and ensuring that it is goal-oriented is a good approach to take when considering how to live your day-to-day life.

Will my thinking here help me avoid conflict with others?

What you might consider to be a conflict may be different than what others might consider to be a conflict. However, with that in mind, significant conflict is what you consider to be above the threshold of the amount you think is acceptable. For example, having an affair and thereby cheating on your spouse is going to cause conflict with others. Being argumentative with your mother-in-law is going to cause conflict with others. Drinking excessively might cause conflict with others. I think this question is simple to understand. If your thinking does not help you avoid conflict with others, especially with someone who has your best interests in mind, it might be best to change this line of thinking.

Will my thinking here help me feel the way I want to feel?

Irrational thinking can contribute (heavily) to how you feel. Ever get rejected by someone you have a crush on? It hurts...of course, right? However, if you are rejected by someone you have a crush on and then tell yourself, "I'm going to be alone forever," that will obviously hurt more. A key component to how your thinking may influence how you feel is if your thinking is hopeless. When people experience depression, as an example, telling yourself, "It will never get better" is a loss of hope. When you are depressed *and* hopeless, things like suicide might seem like a viable option. If you are depressed and you tell yourself, "I can get help, and it will get better," it can instill hope.

Using these five questions can help people who are experiencing negative emotions to challenge their thinking and manage their moods. When you are working to cope with how you feel, challenging your thinking may be beneficial, and it is listed in the appendix as a result.

5. Hobbies/Recreational Activities

This one is so obvious, people often forget about it. Hobbies and recreational activities are closely tied in with the theme of self-care. Recreational activity (unless it is recreational drug use) is almost always good for your emotional well-being. And for the record, work doesn't count as a hobby or recreational activity.

For me (Dr. Walden), my recreational activities are cooking and fishing. Fishing typically involves exercise, because I'm kayak fishing. I can go outside in beautiful Florida with just the birds, wind, waves, and hopefully fish. If all goes as planned, the result is cooking the fresh fish. Cooking requires patience, experience, and continued learning, and there's always a new dish or recipe to make. It engages all five of your senses, allows for creativity, and has successes and failures (such as burned dishes). And best of all, when you are done, you get a meal out of it. For me, these two activities are hobbies that I do multiple times a week—a welcome mental engagement with something that isn't psychotherapy. This mental engagement allows me to recharge, destress, and look forward to the next day when I get to help more people.

If you are struggling to identify a hobby, my suggestion is to ask yourself if there is something you used to enjoy and maybe start there. I can't tell you how often I hear people talk about how much they used to play piano, or paint, or go hunting, but then say they "don't do that anymore." Why not? Most people will report, "I can't because I don't have time," or, "I don't have the money."

We are all busy, and time seems to slip away from all of us. However, engaging in and enjoying a hobby is an investment in yourself. Doing something fun helps you cope with everything else in your life. You must grant yourself permission to enjoy yourself, or else what will all this hard work be good for?

As for money, I'm sure that if you asked 99 percent of the people you and I know "Would you like to make more money?" they would say yes. I get that, there are certain expenses to doing things, and fishing is an example. Rods, reels, line, and bait can all add up and be expensive. But recreational activities can also be very low-cost, or even free. Here in Florida, watching the sunset while sitting on the beach is very low-cost and extremely relaxing. Listening to music (whether radio or playing your old recordings) can be very relaxing. Playing games with loved ones can be very relaxing.

Still having trouble thinking of something? Ask your friends and family what they do for fun and try it, maybe even with them. That's how I started fishing. I loved going fishing with my dad. My mother loves gardening, which is personally not my cup of tea, but we both enjoy cooking and have cooked together. Other people collect stamps or coins, build model replicas of cars or planes, or pursue genealogy, furniture restoration, restoring classic cars, or carpentry; it could be anything.

Well, almost anything. There are things that I would *not* consider a good hobby or recreational activity, watching TV as an example. Watching TV is a passive activity physically and mentally. Physically, you are sitting on your couch or lying in bed and watching TV. Mentally, TV is rarely something with which people are rarely fully engaged; it simply washes over you. Contrast TV with cooking, where you must follow directions, mix ingredients, and observe cooking times. TV is more of a distraction, whereas a good hobby requires mental and emotional engagement. Other distractions include excessive social media use and video games. Hobbies engage your brain, require focus, and provide a pathway to self-esteem.

6. Exercise

The physical benefits of exercise are so numerous. These can include losing or maintaining weight, reduced cardiovascular risk, reduced risk of diabetes, reduced risks of some cancers, improved bone strength, improved balance, and increased chances of longevity (Center for Disease Control, 2018).[3] Most of us know of these benefits, and though it may not be laid out in black-and-white, we all know exercise is good.

What you might not know about is the mental health benefits of exercise. If you have ever started working out consistently, you begin to feel better about yourself. Maybe your clothes fit better, or you're getting compliments at the office, or you just *feel* better. This feeling is separate from the obvious physical benefits, but it is this feeling that keeps people going, at least initially. But if this isn't enough, let's look at some of the research on exercise and mental health.

Recall the GAS response described in Chapter One, where your stress response gets stuck in the "on" position. Even moderate exercise (moderate exertion for ten to fifteen minutes) reduces physiological reactivity to stress.[4] Exercise has also been shown to reduce anxiety, depression, and negative mood, in part by improving self-esteem.[5] Many studies suggest that exercise is as effective in treating depression as medication and psychotherapy.[6] Exercise can also help with fatigue and insomnia. Exercising regularly is known to increase energy during the day. And when it is time to go to sleep, you fall asleep faster and sleep better.[7] Though I would not suggest exercise as a replacement for therapy, I can say confidently that exercise does help people manage negative feelings, and it does so without the potential complications of psychiatric medication.

7. Volunteering

Want to feel better about yourself and help others? Try volunteering. Through volunteering you give something that is truly limited and extremely valuable: your time. Sure, you can donate money. But if you want to make your gift a very real and visceral experience, volunteer your time. I was forced (although I'm thankful that I was now) to volunteer at a homeless shelter as a young boy. I remember complaining about all the things my friends had that I didn't, then I had to go to the local homeless shelter and help serve meals to people who didn't have shoes on their feet. Talk about a wake-up call—it was one that a thirteen-year-old teenager needed. That experience was eye-opening to me and helped me be grateful for the things that I had and less envious of the things that I didn't.

There are volunteer opportunities everywhere. Go to nearly any hospital, animal shelter, library, nursing home, or church and ask. The best thing about volunteering is that you get to help others in need, and to me, that is the greatest gift you can give, and one you can feel good about.

8. Mindfulness

Mindfulness has become extremely popular recently. Mindfulness is derived from Buddhist meditation[8], which emphasizes reaching enlightenment and peace of mind. Mindfulness has been shown to be a helpful technique for depression, anxiety, OCD, addiction, and borderline personality disorder.[9] Why does it work? To put it simply, it is common in our society to slip into autopilot. Watching TV and scrolling through social media are common examples of mind*less* activities. While on autopilot, you may slip into worry about the future (anxiety) or into regret about the past (depression). As a result, the *moment* gets lost.

Mindfulness focuses on living in the moment, fully aware and without judgment. During mindfulness meditation, you are called on to be mindful of when your mind leaves the present moment and then gently return to the present. The present contains physical sensations (what you feel, hear, see, touch, and taste) as well as your thoughts and feelings. Imagine that you are on the ground and that your thoughts are in the sky. You are not reacting to the clouds, merely observing them.

Mindfulness is an especially helpful technique for specific difficulties, such as worry or obsessive thinking (rumination), cravings, and sleep problems. When you ruminate, you are typically thinking about the future. Mindfulness brings you back to the present moment and reduces the anxiety associated with worry. Mindfulness can be helpful in coping with cravings or triggers for addiction. Anyone who's tried to stop smoking has thought, "I need a cigarette right now." Mindfulness reminds us that cravings are merely thoughts that can be observed rather than compelling us to react. The final example is sleep. As soon as you put your head down, you start worrying about tomorrow. Focusing on the moment and what you feel (sheets, pillows) or hear (breathing, AC turning on, ceiling fan) can help bring your mind back to the moment.

There are many mindfulness resources online. Dr. Kabat-Zinn founded the Mindfulness-Based Stress Reduction program at the University of Massachusetts. His book *Wherever You Go, There You Are: Mindfulness Meditation In Everyday Life* is superb.[10] There are also several videos of Dr. Kabat-Zinn on YouTube where you can hear it from the man himself.

9. Get your social black belt.

A book I would recommend to anyone who needs help is *Your Mind, An Owner's Manual for a Better Life*[11] by Drs. Chris Cortman and Harold Shinitzky. The book reviews ten psychological truths which are backed by research and have held true over the course of millennia (and can be seen in biblical texts). The book is also the basis for a social and emotional learning program called the Social Black Belt that is being worked into school districts around the nation.

So what is the point of this book? It helps you prepare for the challenges of everyday living. These truths are universal and are relevant throughout one's lifespan, and if you can live them and understand them, it is extremely beneficial. I (Dr. Walden) frequently cite the ten truths in my therapy sessions because they are easy to digest and help clients understand their own behaviors and others' behaviors.

I'll list what the ten truths are and briefly touch on the significance behind each. The book is available online through Amazon or Barnes and Noble.

Truth #1: Emotions are not mysterious visitors; they can be identified and understood.

People have difficulty understanding their emotions. They have even more difficulty communicating their emotions effectively. Well, I'm here to tell you that emotions have a purpose and are significant. Our emotions are statements about ourselves and are likely the result of our thoughts, attitudes, and beliefs. We are most emotional about the things in which we are most invested. For example, most parents are very invested in their child's health, and if your child hurts, you hurt with them. If you can understand why you feel a certain way, communicating that to another human becomes easier.

Truth #2: You can change your compulsive behaviors if you change your thoughts and address your feelings.

Compulsive behaviors (i.e. denial, avoidance, and substance abuse) are intended to alter how we feel and are usually (temporarily) effective. Compulsive behaviors also tend to continue despite negative consequences, because we all have patterns of behavior. But we can change these harmful behaviors and break the cycle by changing our thoughts about the bad behavior. The bad behavior is an attempt to relieve a negative feeling, but addressing these feelings in a healthier way is a better option.

Truth #3: Every behavior has an underlying purpose, and it's not always what we think.

This truth states that we do *everything* for a reason, and of course, sometimes that reason is not clear or obvious to us. Mr. Avoidance, a pattern we spoke about earlier in this book, is an example of purposeful behavior that might not be obvious to the person. Avoiding talking about a sexual assault that you experienced denies the fact that this terrible thing did happen. The purpose of not talking about it, then, is allowing the individual to pretend that it didn't happen to them. Determining the purpose of the behavior can be extremely helpful in understanding if the behavior is helpful or not.

Truth #4: We all sabotage ourselves unless we confront out internal saboteur.

We have an internal monologue that can be our best friend or our worst enemy. I think the expression, "I'm my own worst critic" speaks to this "internal saboteur." If you've ever thought "I'm my own worst critic," this truth is for you. While the inner saboteur may seem like a friend protecting us from fearful things like rejection, failure, and disappointment, more often than not it prevents us from reaching our potential.

Truth #5: All behavior requires permission, so we must learn what we're permitting ourselves to do.

This truth is related to the concept that you are the only one who gives yourself permission to engage in any behavior. For example, speeding while you're driving doesn't just happen, it occurs because you give yourself permission to drive above the speed limit. We grant ourselves permission to engage in all behavior, good or bad. And if that behavior is unhealthy, removing the permission for the behavior to occur will likely benefit you.

Truth #6: Emotional energy is finite and needs to be invested, rather than wasted on wishing, worrying, and whining.

Everyone wakes up every day with a limited amount of "emotional energy." It's helpful to think about your emotional energy as if it were money. Let's say you wake up every day with $100 worth of energy that you can spend any way you see fit. Let's say you spend $35 on worry, $20 on resentment, and $10 on anger. That leaves you with only $35 left for work, your two kids, your husband, and yourself—not much of a budget. Managing your budget and allotting "money" (emotional energy) for things that will yield a return (such as exercising, date night, or self-care) is the best way to manage your money.

Truth #7: Our relationships depend on self-empowerment and not on enabling others.

Paying bills for your adult child who has careless spending habits is enabling. Picking up a six-pack for your alcoholic mother on your way to her house is enabling. And while this may be easier than arguing with that person, it doesn't make you feel very good. Setting boundaries with others and using assertive communication is a healthier approach.

Truth #8: Ego boundaries protect us from rejection, insult, and intimidation.

An "ego boundary" is the line that separates where you begin and where another person begins. People benefit from being critically aware that they are not responsible for what others say and do. Too often people fall into the trap of thinking, "What did I do wrong?" Having healthy ego boundaries can help prevent rejection, insults, or intimidation.

Truth #9: You can trust people to be who they are, not who you want them to be.

People fall into patterns of behavior, for better or worse. We all have at least one friend who is *always* late. Let's say we invite that person to our birthday party. If we expect that they will show up on time, we'd likely be greatly disappointed. However, knowing that you can trust people to be who they are can help manage our expectations, resulting in improved emotional well-being.

Truth #10: Time doesn't heal pain; we heal ourselves by learning how to let go.

This should sound familiar, and if it doesn't, please refer to the book you're holding. This book is actually an elaboration on the tenth truth. Time passing isn't sufficient to heal from traumatic experiences. But by completing the Fritz, you can heal.

Again, the above is by no means a comprehensive representation of the Social Black Belt, but it is a beginning. These ten truths are relevant to almost every single human interaction that you have ever had and will ever have. And knowing these, I think, provides an extremely helpful set of coping skills.

10. Find your own therapist

Finding a good therapist isn't easy, but I'll try to give you information to expedite the process. Also, I'll go through some of the common questions I hear when people try to find a new therapist as well as how to know if you might benefit from therapy.

When do I need to start therapy, or would I even benefit from psychotherapy? Broadly speaking, everyone could benefit from therapy. The content of this book focuses on very heavy material, but even those without trauma may benefit from therapy. Difficulties with your spouse or children, transitions in life (new job, retirement, moving, etc.), insomnia, or addictions are all common reasons to seek therapy. The positive psychology movement has taught us that normal functioning is not necessarily optimal functioning. Everyone deserves to make the most of their life.

When to start? In an ideal world, people would come to therapy before the stage of full-blown depression and suicidality or before full-blown addiction. But often, psychotherapy is a last-ditch option. This is fairly normal, and new clients are frequently in crisis mode. Ideally, however, people come in before they reach rock bottom. If you have ever thought, "Maybe I need to talk to someone about this," then you're probably right. If you feel like you've tried everything, asked friends and family for help, done some internet research on "how to cope with _____," tried medications, and you still remain unhappy, maybe therapy is the answer. In other words, use your emotional well-being (or rather, lack of well-being) as your guide for when to start therapy.

Where to start therapy? The answer depends on your circumstances. First, let's assume you have insurance that covers mental health services. Take out your insurance card. Call your insurer and ask for local, in-network mental health providers. Or try finding a list of local in-network providers on your insurance company's website. This is a kind of a "top-down" approach, in that your insurance company dictates your options for therapists in the area.

The "bottom up" approach is to search Google.com for psychologists in your county. You can call these offices directly and give them your insurance information, and they will determine your cost, co-pay, and whether the therapist is in-network as regards your insurance. PsychologyToday.com allows you to search by city or zip code. After this search, you can refine your results with more filter options, including insurance providers accepted, gender, languages spoken, type of issues, and so on. These can help narrow the search for someone with whom you'll feel comfortable. If you click on a therapist link, there's usually a photo and a brief description, along with credentials, areas of expertise, and contact information.

Who should you pick? I often hear, "I only want to see a PhD" and, "Are mental health counselors good enough?" There are some excellent masters-level counselors out there, and some really horrible doctors. Consider experience with specific issues. Someone with a master's degree who has worked with children for fifteen years is going to do better with children than a psychologist who has specialized in addictions. Training and experience trump credentials.

Another question I hear often is, "Should I work with a male or female therapist?" Success in therapy depends heavily on the relationship with your therapist, so choose someone you're likely to be most comfortable opening up to emotionally. Here's something else to think about, though: to use an example, being a male psychologist working with females who have been traumatized by men provides certain challenges and benefits. Of course, after learning a female client of mine has been victimized in some way by a man, my job is to help her feel safe and trust me in the early sessions. Having this experience can in and of itself be therapeutic. Learning to feel safe and trust someone who resembles the individual(s) who created your issues is probably helpful.

Regardless of who you pick, you should feel confident in this person's abilities, feel better, feel more hopeful, and look forward to working together. If you don't feel this way within the first two sessions, find another therapist. I've heard stories of people staying in therapy with someone for months, or sometimes years, with someone with whom they don't feel comfortable or who is not benefiting them. This is very frustrating indeed. If you are sitting there and have questions, comments, or concerns, share these with your therapist. It's called talk therapy for a reason. If you're not sure about the direction of therapy, ask them. Communication is the foundation on which a strong therapeutic relationship is built, so communicate openly and freely. The therapeutic relationship is unique and different from any other relationship, so if you don't feel helped quickly, don't wait around for it to improve. If you're at a private practice where there are other counselors, ask to see a different counselor, or if you must, find a new office altogether. Hopefully, you won't have to do this too many times before you find someone who you believe you can work with.

I want therapy, but I don't have insurance and can't afford it. Many Americans don't have insurance, but still want help. Most offices have a self-pay rate offered to people who don't have insurance or who don't want to use their insurance. Call different offices and find out what these rates are and determine if you can afford them. Most offices also have a sliding scale rate which considers your income and adjusts the self-pay rate accordingly. Again, you must call and ask. Also note that the average Master's-level counselor charges less than the average psychologist., and there are excellent Master's-level therapists out there. Some offices have students in training who are close to completing their graduate degree and can still provide excellent therapy.

If you find a therapist you really think will be perfect for you, but their rate for a session is steep, try seeing that person at a reduced frequency. Typically, with insurance companies, seeing a therapist once a week is standard, however if you're paying out of pocket, attending treatment every other week, or even once a month, may be cost-effective.

Some treatment facilities are funded by the state or county and are more affordable. This includes community mental health hospitals. These facilities often offer group therapy, which can be very affordable. There is the discomfort of sharing your issues with a group, but you also receive feedback and encouragement from multiple people, not just a therapist, and this feedback can be quite helpful.

In sum, cost is a very real concern, but thinking that you can't afford therapy often prevents people from getting help they really need. Certainly cost is important, but so is your mental well-being. So, call private practices and community mental health centers and see what you can work out. Not having insurance makes receiving services a bit more challenging and does require more legwork, but there are still options out there if you persevere.

References: Appendix Two

1. W., Bill. (1976). *Alcoholics Anonymous: The Story of How Many Thousands of Men and Women Have Recovered From Alcoholism.* New York, NY: Alcoholics Anonymous World Services.

2. Patton, P., L. (1992). Rational Behavior Training: A Seven Lesson Sequence for Teaching Rational Behavioral Skills to Students with Social and Emotional Disabilities. Retrieved from https://files.eric.ed.gov/fulltext/ED350807.pdf

3. Center for Disease Control. (2018). *Physical Activity and Health.* Atlanta, GA: Retrieved from https://www.cdc.gov/physicalactivity/basics/pa-health/index.htm

4. Sharma, A., Madaan, V., & Petty, F. D. (2006). Exercise for Mental Health. *Primary Care Companion to The Journal of Clinical Psychiatry, 8*(2), 106.

5. Callaghan, P. (2004). Exercise: a neglected intervention in mental health care? *Journal of Psychiatric and Mental Health Nursing, 11*, 476-483.

6. Blumenthal, J. A., Smith, P. J., & Hoffman, B. M. (2012). Is Exercise a Viable Treatment for Depression? *ACSM's Health & Fitness Journal, 16*(4), 14–21.

7. Strauss Cohen, I. (2017). 7 Unexpected Mental Health Benefits of Exercising. *Psych Central.* Retrieved on June 12, 2018, from https://psychcentral.com/blog/7-unexpected-mental-health-benefits-of-exercising/

8. Fossas, A. (2015). *The Basics of Mindfulness: Where did it come from?* Retrieved from https://welldoing.org/article/basics-of-mindfulness-come-from

9.   Henriques, G. (2015) *What is Mindfulness and How Does It Work?* Retrieved from https://www.psychologytoday.com/us/blog/theory-knowledge/201502/what-is-mindfulness-and-how-does-it-work

10.   Kabat-Zinn, Jon. (1994). *Wherever You Go, There You Are: Mindfulness Meditation In Everyday Life*. New York, NY: Hyperion.

11.   Cortman, C., Shinitzky, H. (2010). *Your Mind: An Owner's Manual For A Better Life*. Franklin Lakes, NJ: Career Press.

Acknowledgments

In the words of Nelson Mandela, "Courage is not the absence of fear, but the triumph over it. The brave man is not he who does not feel afraid, but he who conquers that fear."

I'll begin my list of acknowledgments with the bravest person I know personally, my wife, Stephanie, who is raising three children and a childish husband, all while grappling with stage four breast cancer. Thank you, Steph, for supporting me through yet another book. Maybe I'll write the next one on "How to become the perfect husband."

Thank you also to my children, Cameron, Melina, and Dylan for sacrificing "Daddy time" so I could work on this project. I promise I'll never do this again until mommy says it's time to write another book.

Much gratitude to our literary agent, Giles Anderson, who believed in the project right from the outset and sought to find the perfect publishing company. I'd like to also thank that perfect publishing company, Mango Publishing, especially Brenda Knight, a woman with the personality to make you think that you are doing things out of your own free will, when in fact, you are actually under her spell. Although we have never met, I'd like to thank you for your patience with us and your ability to find laughter in every situation. And although we may have contributed to your desire to opt for an early retirement, I would work with you again without reservation!

A word of gratitude to my brave "work wives," Lexi and Smeather. I salute you for your daily patience and your long suffering with me, exacerbated by the deadline of publishing a book. I appreciate your encouragement, kindness, and consistency. There, that's better than a raise any day! No?

To my co-author, Dr. Joseph Walden, thank you for your many insights and contributions to this book. May you enjoy a long career that is every bit as fantastic as you are.

A heartfelt thank you to Bruce, my extraordinary editor, and Dr. Roger Davis, my unpaid but brilliant psychologist editor. You are a gentleman and a true friend!

My thanks to Fritz Perls, Albert Ellis, David Burns, Donald Michenbaum, Lenore Terr, Syd Simon, Charles Whitfield, Judith Herman, Robert Ackerman, Martin Seligman, E. Sue Blume, and so many other psychologists and mental health professionals who have contributed to my knowledge in treating patients with trauma, grief and "unfinished business".

Most importantly, I tip my hat to the scores of broken people who have allowed me into their lives to help them recover from the worst of what life has to offer. Don't tell the above psychologists, but you all have taught me more about how the mind heals than all of the psychologists combined. I am grateful to you, my teachers/students for helping me to put together a paradigm for treatment that truly works. May you always feel the joy of contributing to the healing of others. God bless each one of you for your remarkable recovery, continued courage, and faith moving forward. To each of you, you humble and inspire me.

CHRISTOPHER CORTMAN

I'll begin my acknowledgments with the person who got me interested in the field in the first place and pushed me (sometimes kicking and screaming) into pursuing my doctorate, my dad. Though you are no longer here in person, your influence on my life has been undeniable, and I know you're looking down on me and that you are proud. My mom has been my biggest supporter of late and has encouraged me to strive for excellence. Without her strength over the past few years, none of this, including working on this book, would have been possible.

To my fiancé, Tricia, you are the sunshine in my life and have been throughout our relationship. Whenever I need support, you've been there, and while writing this book, it was no different. I am looking forward to marrying you and am excited for our wedding and our future together.

To my supervisor, colleague, and friend Chris Cortman, I am truly blessed to have the opportunity to work for, learn from, and write this book with you. The wisdom I've been able to absorb from someone who has run a successful practice for thirty years and has helped thousands of people will be put to good use throughout my career in the near and distant future. Not many people get to publish a book in their twenties, but with your help I have gotten there, and I couldn't be more thankful.

I'd also like to thank Dr. Roger Davis for his knowledge and excellent editorial skills and Jessica Reyka for selflessly giving me this opportunity to work on the book.

As mentioned above, a big thank-you to the clients who have worked so hard with me to heal from the worse experiences known to man. And a special thank-you to our veterans, because war truly is Hell, and healing from it is challenging. To all the people I've worked with, I am always in awe of your resilience, and your continued strength motivates me to be the best psychologist I can be. The journeys that you have gone through with treatment are daunting at times, but the healing that can occur is so profound it helps me stay grounded, stay humble, and stay motivated to help more and more people.

JOSEPH WALDEN

About the Authors

Joseph Walden

Dr. Joseph Walden graduated from Florida State University with his Bachelor's degree in psychology and graduated with his Doctorate of Psychology from the Florida School of Professional Psychology. Dr. Walden has a wide variety of experiences including working in a crisis center and an inpatient drug and alcohol center in Bradenton, a college counseling center in and the C.W. Bill Young VA Medical Center in St. Petersburg, and Park Center, a community mental health hospital, in Fort Wayne, Indiana. Dr. Walden has worked with children, families, adults, and the geriatric populations in individual and group therapy. He offers treatment for anxiety, depression, addictions, trauma, interpersonal skills, phobias, and stress management. "I am personally and professionally invested in the treatment of the military population. My father was an Army veteran and was the one who originally sparked my interest in the treatment of trauma. While on practicum at the Bay Pines VAMC, I worked in the Substance and Posttraumatic Integrated Recovery (SPIR) unit where I worked with veterans who were dually diagnosed with an alcohol/drug addiction and PTSD. There I spent time completing trauma-specific training for my entire tenure there. I also completed my dissertation using an empirical study regarding differences in PTSD symptom expression across war era involvement."

Christopher Cortman

Chris Cortman, PhD has been a licensed psychologist for 28 years. He is a much-sought-after speaker, has facilitated more than 60,000 hours of psychotherapy, and has provided psychological consultation at five hospitals in the Sarasota/Venice area. Dr. Cortman is the co-creator of a youth prevention and wellness program called The Social Black Belt.

Printed in the USA
CPSIA information can be obtained
at www.ICGtesting.com
JSHW031704140824
68134JS00036B/3513